Successful Supervision in Health Care Practice

Promoting Professional Development

Edited by

Jenny Spouse and Liz Redfern

b

**Blackwell
Science**

© 2000 by
Blackwell Science Ltd
Editorial Offices:
Osney Mead, Oxford OX2 0EL
25 John Street, London WC1N 2BL
23 Ainslie Place, Edinburgh EH3 6AJ
350 Main Street, Malden
  MA 02148 5018, USA
54 University Street, Carlton
  Victoria 3053, Australia
10, rue Casimir Delavigne
  75006 Paris, France

Other Editorial Offices:

Blackwell Wissenschafts-Verlag GmbH
Kurfürstendamm 57
10707 Berlin, Germany

Blackwell Science KK
MG Kodenmacho Building
7–10 Kodenmacho Nihombashi
Chuo-ku, Tokyo 104, Japan

First published 2000

Set in 10/12.5 pt Sabon
by DP Photosetting, Aylesbury, Bucks
Printed and bound in Great Britain by
MPG Books, Bodmin, Cornwall

DISTRIBUTORS

Marston Book Services Ltd
PO Box 269
Abingdon
Oxon OX14 4YN
(Orders: Tel: 01235 465500
          Fax: 01235 465555)

USA
Blackwell Science, Inc.
Commerce Place
350 Main Street
Malden, MA 02148 5018
(Orders: Tel: 800 759 6102
               781 388 8250
          Fax: 781 388 8255)

Canada
Login Brothers Book Company
324 Saulteaux Crescent
Winnipeg, Manitoba R3J 3T2
(Orders: Tel: 204 837 2987
          Fax: 204 837 3116)

Australia
Blackwell Science Pty Ltd
54 University Street
Carlton, Victoria 3053
(Orders: Tel: 03 9347 0300
          Fax: 03 9347 5001)

A catalogue record for this title is available
from the British Library

ISBN 0-632-05159-0

Library of Congress
Cataloging-in-Publication Data
Successful supervision in health care
  practice/edited by Jenny Spouse and
  Liz Redfern.
    p. cm.
    Includes bibliographical references and
index.
    ISBN 0-632-05159-0 (pbk.)
    1. Medical personnel–In-service
training. 2. Mentoring in medicine.
3. Medicine–Study and teaching–
Supervision.
I. Spouse, Jenny. II. Redfern, Liz.
R834.S87   1999
610'.71'55–dc21
                              99-38176
                                   CIP

For further information on
Blackwell Science, visit our website:
www.blackwell-science.com

Contents

Contributors

Sally Ballard BA (Hons) Nursing, RN   Sally took a 4-year nursing degree at Oxford Brookes University, registering as an adult nurse in 1995. Since then she has worked as a staff nurse in wards concerned with rehabilitation of older persons, in neurosurgical nursing and most recently in a general surgical nursing ward of her local hospital. She is currently completing a part-time certificate in adult education and has just been appointed clinical nursing skills teacher at Oxford Brookes University.

Lisa M. Benrud-Larson PhD   Lisa earned a BA in psychology from Luther College in Decorah, Iowa, and an MS and PhD in clinical psychology from the University of Wisconsin-Milwaukee. She is currently a postdoctoral fellow in the Department of Psychiatry and Behavioral Sciences at Johns Hopkins University in Baltimore, Maryland.

Charlotte Chesson BSc (Hons), RGN, FETC, PgDipProfessional Ed, PgDipAdvanced Health Care Practice   Charlotte works as a tutor/facilitator within 'The Learning Curve' Oxfordshire Mental Healthcare Trust, formerly known as Oxfordshire Clinical Education and Practice Team. Prior to this post she was an 'F' grade staff nurse and team leader within the area of acute medicine.

Lorna Cowan RN, RM, MPublic Health, PgDipProfessional Ed   Until recently Lorna was working as a community midwife in Oxfordshire. Previously she worked as an independent midwife, a team midwife and a lecturer/practitioner midwife. She has recently commenced a new appointment as a practice development midwife in the delivery suite on a job-share basis at the Oxford Radcliffe Trust in Oxfordshire.

Ann Davies BA (Hons), Dip OTCot, SROT   Ann trained as an occupational therapist at York, graduating in 1978. Much of her career has been in mental health. She has been head occupational therapist at Bolton NHS Trust for 13 years. She has a degree in English Literature from Manchester University for which she studied part-time, graduating in 1996.

Louise Dumas RN, BScInf., MSN, PhD   Louise is a clinical nurse specialist, and is professor-researcher in nursing sciences at the University of Quebec at Hull, Canada. She is also adjunct professor to the MNursing Sciences at the University of Ottawa (Ontario). Her main teaching and research interests are perinatal nursing; teaching and learning related to health professionals; and patient teaching.

Janet Gregson Dip COT, SROT   Janet is a senior occupational therapist in mental health with Bolton NHS Trust. After a career break Janet returned to work in a large general hospital, initially working part time with the older adult, and has since moved to working with adults suffering from acute mental health problems. In August 1998 she moved to work full time in a multi-disciplinary community mental health team. She has a special interest in counselling and inter-agency working and is currently collaborating with the local adult education service in group work for people with mental health problems.

Claire- Louise Hatton   Claire-Louise first qualified in 1988 in acupuncture at the College of Traditional Acupuncture, Leamington Spa (England). She joined the teaching faculty at the College in 1993 and received her Acupuncture Masters in 1997. Claire-Louise teaches clinical year students and is a member of the postgraduate studies team. She has a private practice in Oxford.

Mary Kavanagh Dip COT, MSc   Mary is a lecturer/practitioner (occupational therapy) at Oxford Brookes University and works for a community mental health team. She has wide clinical experience of working with people suffering from acute mental and physical health problems, including addiction. She has a specific interest in group-work training skills for assertiveness and anxiety management.

Krysia Lewandowski DCR Diagnostic Radiography, ARRT, Clinical Teaching Certificate, FAETC, BSc(Hons)Psychology   Having worked in clinical practice in a large teaching hospital for four years Krysia became a Clinical Teacher for radiography students. She continues to work with both undergraduates and postgraduate clinical staff as a Clinical Training Coordinator. Her interests are in communication and interpersonal skills, and running short courses and workshops for clinical personnel. Her research interests are in levels of expertise in clinical practice.

Barbara Lovelady RGN, BSc (Hons), PgDipProfessional Ed, MSc   Barbara is working as clinical lecturer based in a general intensive care unit and teaching on pre- and post-registration degree programmes. She has extensive cardiac critical care experience both in England and Australia and originally trained in London, qualifying in 1989. She has always had a keen interest in teaching and learning in the clinical environment.

Nigel Northcott PhD, MA(Ed), RGN, PGCEA, Dip(N) Nigel is an independent professional consultant educator who uses his extensive experience of working with health care staff to assist them to extend and develop their potential. He is currently engaged in a number of research projects associated with narrative evaluation of health care experience, and teaches on a masters degree in nursing.

Liz Redfern BEd (Hons), RGN, RSCN, RCNT, RNT, DipCounselling & Therapy Liz has a background in nursing and nursing education and has held a number of senior positions in colleges of nursing and midwifery. She was Assistant Director for Educational Policy (Continuing Education) at the English National Board for Nursing, Midwifery and Health Visiting before establishing her own business, working as an organisational and personal development consultant with clients from the field of health care. She is an advisory editor to the *Nursing Times* and editor of *Learning Curve*. She is also a non-executive director of Northamptonshire Health Authority and Joint Regional Director of Nursing for the South-West NHS Executive.

Dave Roberts MSc, RMN, RGN Dave is a clinical nurse specialist in mental health at the John Radcliffe Hospital in Oxford. He is also a member of the Oxford Psycho-Oncology Service and visiting lecturer at Oxford Brookes University. He is secretary to the Royal College of Nursing special interest group in liaison mental health nursing.

David Robson MB, BS, FRCP David is a consultant physician at Greenwich Hospital. His clinical special interests are cardiology and intensive care. He was director of the Greenwich Hospital Support System Project and subsequently Service Director for Medicine and the Service Director for Information. Currently he is Head of Information Strategy and Clinical Systems for Greenwich Healthcare Trust. These roles have involved management of service and training budgets for clinical staff, development strategies to support improvements in patient care and to prepare for the introduction of clinical governance.

Lesley Rudd MSc, RN, MIPD, MHSM Lesley is Chief Nurse/Director of Quality at Barnet Healthcare NHS Trust, and Designate Joint Regional Director of Nursing for the South West NHS Executive. Since training as a nurse she has worked in health, education and counselling, and personnel/ development management. She has been a sister in oncology services as well as doing clinical work in general paediatrics, cardiology and the community. Lesley has been a director in the National Health Service for over six years, covering the whole range of acute, community, mental health, learning disability and specialist services. Her interest in clinical supervision began when she was a counsellor in the late 1970s. Since then she has made it part of her work to implement and introduce good supervision with the need to improve patient care.

Paul Simic BA (Hons), CQSW, DipPSW, MSc   Paul is director of the Applied Research and Consultancy Centre in the Department of Social Policy and Social Work at Manchester University. He has written on a range of subjects but has a particular interest in joint working between health and social services.

Jenny Spouse PhD, MSc, RN, RM, RCNT, RNT   Jenny is a lecturer in work-based learning at the Open University. She has worked as a nurse in a range of clinical settings in the UK as well as in Canada and Australia. Her interests are concerned with the professional development of pre- and post-registration practitioners and particularly with the quality of the learning environment in clinical settings.

Philip Wolsey   Phil has a mental health background and worked in the NHS for 20 years as a practitioner, manager and lecturer-practitioner. He holds a masters degree in mental health and qualifications in nursing, social work and teaching. He is now a Certified Management Consultant and Senior Partner in the Consultancy, OPDC.

Preface

Recognition of learning and professional development as life long activities has highlighted the need for strategies to enable such personal growth in every health care practitioner. It requires significant financial and personal commitment from all those involved at every level of a health care organisation. Much of this interest has been fuelled by public concern at the quality of care available in public and private sectors of health care provision. Resources for staff development vary and their effective use is often difficult to demonstrate.

The largest group of practitioners in health care settings is nurses. It is inevitable that recent public attention has been directed to the adequacy of their preparation. The problems nurses face when learning in busy clinical environments are also shared by students from every other profession involved in health care delivery. Such difficulties do not go away following qualification. With rapid changes in technology and increased understanding of health and disease, pressures are ever present to maintain and further develop professional knowledge and practice.

These demands are increasingly acknowledged by governmental and professional bodies that are now introducing the necessary structures for forms of supervision tailored to meet career needs at different stages in a professional's life. The flurry of texts explaining the value of supervision in all these forms demonstrates the seriousness with which health care professionals are addressing such demands. These tend to offer academically orientated commentaries on the value and importance of clinical supervision or of mentorship. Others provide accounts written by managers and practitioners of how they have introduced supervision to their clinical setting. They provide valuable insights to how professions such as social work and health visiting use supervision but they often lack the human perspective of the supervision process. Yet others provide excellent guidance to nurses wishing to develop their skills of clinical supervision, and give a wealth of well-reasoned, practical activities supported by relevant literature based on extensive experience of personal supervision and of preparing practitioners to be supervisors.

From reviewing this range of literature, there seemed to be a need for a more human account of what it is like to be a supervisor – a need to walk in the same shoes of supervisors working in clinical practice and wrestling with all the demands that it imposes, whilst also being mindful of the needs of colleagues, or to walk in the shoes of a student trying to learn and work effectively. This need raised further questions such as: how does a practitioner manage such demands and what are the issues he or she faces? How can supervision and assessment or appraisal go together and what is their relationship? What do you do if you are a specialist and there is no one else within reach who has the same experiences?

Rationale for the book

The available research indicates that supervision is being introduced in a range of settings, but that its effectiveness is difficult to determine. Accounts suggest that much depends upon the relationship between supervisor and supervisee and the influence of external pressures upon the relationship. By taking a critical theory approach, this book uses the principles of action inquiry and reflective practice (Zuber-Skerrit 1992; Boud *et al.* 1985) and seeks to provide practitioners with a means to strengthen their own voice (Belenky *et al.* 1986) whilst supporting their own professional development and that of their colleagues (Daloz 1986).

Most practitioners have an abiding interest in people and how they cope with experience. We have compiled this book to give a multi-professional perspective on what it is like to be a supervisor and to cope with a whole range of common practical and professional problems. Contributors all work as supervisors in a range of institutional and community settings and give supervision to colleagues at different stages of their career. With increasing recognition that students need effective support and education in clinical settings there are rather more accounts from practitioners concerned with student preparation. Some supervisors work in professions supplementary to medicine and others as complimentary therapists. They have all created reflective accounts of critical incidents that helped them gain greater insight into their role with the hope that readers will benefit from their experiences. To supplement these accounts there are two descriptions of experiences of good supervision written by students, one a nurse and the other a clinical psychologist. Other accounts are from practitioners and managers who are either working with colleagues to provide effective professional support or who have set up structures and processes for supervision to be used in their Trust.

These scenarios are supplemented by material from two different research studies. The first is concerned with exploring practitioners' understanding and experiences of appraisal and its relationship to supervision. From this study some valuable issues concerned with management style and communication are raised. The discussion will be particularly helpful to practitioners wishing to introduce both activities in their setting or to increase their understanding.

The second research study is concerned with the professional development of students and factors influencing their development. Good mentorship was found to be the most vital factor to student development. From this research evidence a five-part model has been developed and this is presented and discussed. Although the research is concerned with student supervision, subsequent work indicates that it has relevance to everyone who provides supervision of any sort. Supporting this material is a chapter describing a curriculum used to prepare health care practitioners to become supervisors. The processes can be used in a range of clinical settings as well as classrooms, irrespective of the number of people involved, and so has relevance for practitioners and teachers alike.

Notes to the reader

Learning how to supervise a colleague, whether a peer or a student, is a dynamic and unique process. Each one of us seeks to find ways that reflects our personality, our relationship with our colleague and the setting. Although some basic suggestions are made in the models we are offering, they will inevitably need to be adapted to your own situation. The same applies to our contributors' accounts. Written as reflective accounts by novice and experienced supervisors they provide hope and encouragement to practitioners whilst offering scenarios for discussion and role-play in different settings. Contributors' solutions to the problems they faced reflect their best knowledge at the time and are personal solutions rather than recipes for an audience. As a result you may find that you disagree with an approach that has been described but we hope it will stimulate ideas for finding your own solutions.

We would welcome your feedback and contributions. This would help us share experiences that reflect the challenges and successes of our different professions, and experience what it is like to truly participate in a community of practice. When preparing this book we believed it to be important to maintain an informal style so we did not impose a rigid framework on each of the contributions. Each writer has used a style that reflects his or her particular approach. Because these are largely personal accounts or based on research data, they reflect the gender of the participants rather than an anonymous being.

Jenny Spouse and Liz Redfern

References

Belenky, M.F., Clinchy, M.B., Goldberg, N.R. & Tarule, J.M. (1986) *Women's Ways of Knowing: The Development of Self, Voice and Mind*. Basic Books, New York.

Boud, D., Keough, R. & Walker, D. (1985) *Reflection: Turning Experience into Learning*. Kogan Page, London.

Daloz, L.A. (1986) *Effective Teaching and Mentoring*. Jossey Bass, San Francisco.

Zuber-Skerrit, O. (1992) *Action Research in Higher Education: Examples and Reflections*. Kogan Page, London.

Chapter 1

Creating a Quality Service

Jenny Spouse and Liz Redfern

Rapid developments in technology and the expansion of health care options counterbalanced by rising costs and demographic changes have forced governments to review their approach to health care provision. Quality has become a significant part of the health care agenda, placing consumers at the centre of attention with the workforce some way behind in second place. The philosophical basis for successful service provision must be based on quality. Quality must be designed into structures that will provide suitable conditions for staff to work effectively and efficiently. Structures must also be established that ensure staff are educated and prepared to meet continuing demands of changing technology and health care requirements. Without these physical, social and educational structures, reforms instituted by professional statutory bodies and governments will fail to manage escalating health care costs and will fail to recruit and retain staff (Ovretveit 1992).

Starting with the paper *Working for Patients* (Department of Health 1989), government reforms have continued to focus attention on improving services by increasing consumer (patient) involvement in setting standards of health care at local levels and by increasing professional accountability through clinical governance (Department of Health 1991). These reforms have continued with further government initiatives, and publications such as *A First Class Service – Quality in the New NHS* (DoH 1998) that endorse the importance of quality values and approaches. Further government initiatives are concerned with developing human resources within health and social care to create a force of skilled and highly motivated staff. Policies must take account of professional practice and build upon earlier directives aimed at improving care. These initiatives have significant implications for health care providers who must implement and monitor their effectiveness. Health care providers have a responsibility to conserve resources effectively and this is a greater responsibility than managing problems when they arise. They must find ways of ensuring that problems do not arise by systematically monitoring practice and instituting changes. Providing a quality service means ensuring staff are knowledgeable and skilled in the range of techniques necessary to carry out care. This includes assessing need, being able to provide care, and using techniques and knowledge properly. Effective supervision is also needed to support and to give guidance to practitioners (Ovretveit 1992). Implicit in such expectations is the provision of suitable conditions for health care practice to take place. Such conditions must include suitable working environments and equipment as well as provision of adequate numbers of staff able to carry out the work effectively and efficiently (Donabedian 1966). In exchange, professionals are expected to maintain and develop their professional knowledge so that they continue to be fit to practise safely and effectively. Professional statutory organisations have responsibility for protecting the public by developing professional standards of performance and for ensuring that they are maintained. None of this can take place effectively without full collaboration from all the participants. Quality health care can only be achieved when statutory bodies, health care providers and practitioners work together, each ensuring that the other receives the maximum support.

Professional development

Development is concerned with individual personal growth. It deals with feeling and thinking and practical application to life activities. This definition uses a more holistic form of learning involving personal and interpersonal skills such as problem solving, initiative, efficiency, and interactional and communication skills. Professional development moves this person-centred approach towards a more sophisticated level of incorporating knowledge, skills and attitudes necessary for effective practice. It prepares individuals to work in environments that are uncertain and are changing rapidly. It helps people to develop skills that can be used in a range of settings both at home and at work. They are the skills that enable practitioners to be self-directed, to take the initiative, to work with others, to communicate clearly, to take informed but calculated risks, to make judgements, to be responsible and assertive. These characteristics describe empowered human beings and the way professionals are expected to act.

Professional practice is a dynamic activity that reflects individual encounters. Patient conditions and problems may bear similar characteristics but individuals do not. Thus the idiosyncratic nature of health care practice is its fascination and also its downfall. The fascination of health care is the need to be continuously alert to what patients are saying and experiencing, and to find approaches that will resolve their dis-ease. This requires a complex range of professional skills and knowledge that marries both science and art in skilful, expert practice. Such expertise takes years to accumulate and cannot be acquired after a few years' training and education. Both opera singers and athletes are acknowledged to need a minimum of eight to ten years to reach their peak of performance. Ericsson and his colleagues found that complex skills require repeated exposure and feedback to enable practitioners to improve their performance and concluded that it took an average of ten years to become an expert (Ericsson *et al.* 1993). Ovretveit's (1992) arguments that practitioners need the necessary professional knowledge and skills to be effective carries a message that such knowledge is not static but needs refreshment and development on a continuous basis. It also assumes that practitioners have undertaken sufficient preparation for their role to be effective; to be able to learn continuously and to recognise their own limitations. This continuous development of professional knowledge and understanding can only be effective under guidance and support from more experienced colleagues. Students entering professional practice need to learn in a culture that values education as an essential process rather than seeing it as a luxury or a bonus. Learning and continuous development need to be an accepted part of the fabric of an organisation and built into its policies and procedures. The rapid pace of technological development means knowledge quickly becomes outdated. This was a key concern of the Dearing Report (National Committee of Inquiry into Higher Education 1997). It emphasised the need for high quality education that supports learning as a lifelong process. Every member of the workforce must develop skills to maintain and develop their professional knowledge. Unless this is achieved, practice becomes ritualised and ineffective (Walsh & Ford 1989). Recognition of the importance of affective and practical or experiential knowledge has grown with increasing research into learning and exposure to multicultural approaches to learning. As a result learning in workplace settings has become valued and the role of a supervisor or colleague able to facilitate learning has become increasingly important.

Supervision

'A formal process of professional support and learning which enables individual practitioners to develop knowledge and competence, assume responsibility for their own practice and enhance consumer protection and safety of care in complex clinical situations.' (Department of Health 1993)

Supervision as described in these terms has a distinct quality focus that places education alongside other strategies for quality assurance. Approaches to supervision for professional development vary amongst individual practitioners. This difference could depend upon a range of factors, including personal preferences, the clinical context of work and the professional needs of supervisees. We believe the particular strength of this book lies in Chapters 3 and 4, because they create a window into the real world of supervision, one that works with the theories, history, politics and policies that the remainder of the book describes and debates.

Organisation of the chapters

The chapters of this book relate to each other by exploring different issues that can influence the successful introduction of supervision in professional practice. Some chapters have been written with the authority of empirical research whilst others provide data for research, being first-hand accounts of work and experiences of practitioners in the field. Other chapters discuss this information, conceptualising supervision as a personal process that requires skill and courage as well as preparation and continuing development in itself. The final chapter explores the implications for health care organisations if they are to be effective in ensuring that professional development can take place through supervision.

In collating the chapters of the book we adopted a structure that seeks to address questions such as: Why is supervision such an issue in professional health care? What is the difference between supervision and appraisal? What is supervision and what makes a good supervisor? What sort of things do I need to know when offering supervision? How can a system of supervision be introduced in an under-resourced service? How do I develop skills of supervision in my staff? What are the political and professional implications of supervision?

This introduction has sought to address the first question and to explain the importance of effective professional development and the value of supervision in professional health care. Chapter 2 will explore the differences between supervision and appraisal and provide some definitions of the terms in current use. In particular Nigel Northcott addresses the suspicions that many practitioners have expressed about clinical supervision, confusing its intentions with performance review and appraisal. Nigel Northcott's chapter leads on from his research in this area and clarifies the two processes. He shows how they can complement each other whilst fulfilling distinctively different functions in achieving a quality service. He also adds some warnings about using either approach ineffectively or inappropriately.

The following two chapters provide first-hand accounts of supervision from a variety of perspectives. In doing so they address questions about the nature of good supervision and how it can be implemented.

Chapter 3 contains critical incidents written by eight health care practitioners recounting their experiences of offering supervision in a range of professional settings. They provide courageous insights into the difficulties and challenges that many practitioners experience when trying to address different aspects of the supervisory role. These reflective accounts review issues of teaching skills in clinical settings; the nature of the interpersonal relationship; the qualities of artistry in practice and the fears that often accompany a necessity to challenge and confront dysfunctional behaviour. Such difficulties are probably familiar at some stage in their practice to most mentors, preceptors and supervisors. By exploring their own personal fears and strategies these practitioners provide gifts for readers facing similar challenges. Chapter 3 concludes with accounts written by two students who describe exemplary experiences of supervision. Inherent in all these narratives is evidence of how complex is the supervision process and the stress that it can cause to thoughtful practitioners, particularly in the early stages of learning how to supervise others successfully.

A second significant factor arising from these narratives is the value of reflective practice. The original purpose of this book was to provide illustrations of supervisory activities. We asked contributors to use a framework for analysing their experiences and offered them some models to consider. We had not intended to provide a vehicle for trumpeting reflective practice. But as the accounts came in we were overwhelmed by their honesty, by the personal and professional progress that writers had achieved and by the progress they had demonstrated in their narratives. Such progress has been made with some personal cost and pain. Their growth did not necessarily take place immediately around the event but some time later following discussion and writing about their experience. Most contributors indicate that they are describing an event that took place at least a year before they wrote it up. This is characteristic of reflective practice, and this will be discussed in more detail in Chapter 6. Some of these practitioners used a specific model of reflection to provide hooks around which to frame their discussion, whilst others have been less overt in the model that they have used. An example is the critical incident discussed by French Canadian nurse Louise Dumas (Chapter 3.8), who has developed a supervisory framework based on work by Kolb (1984). She uses this to illustrate a supervisory process between a clinical teacher and a post-registration student who, having practised for eight years, decided to return to study in order to seek promotion. This will be a familiar experience to many clinical educators and supervisors who support professionals returning to education after many years of practice or who are returning to practice after many years away from it, bringing up their family or engaged in other life activities. Several of the accounts are concerned with supporting novices whilst the writers were developing their own professional knowledge. This is a common experience in professions that do not retain practitioners for longer than three or four years. Other contributors write from considerable experience and are concerned with different issues in the supervisory process that reflect their expertise. All have used a simple basic framework in their accounts that encouraged a deeper, more analytical approach to be achieved. This framework comprised:

- A description of the event and the context
- Analysis of what took place
- Exploration of the implications for personal practice

A more detailed discussion of these frameworks will be explored in Chapter 7.

Chapter 4 provides two examples of supervision from an organisational perspective. The first account is a case study of two occupational therapists, Ann Davies and Janet Gregson. They describe their experiences of supervision whilst trying to create a new community service that was multiprofessional. The scale of change that they describe is smaller than that in the subsequent section, but their account is invaluable as it charts many of the issues that can arise in supervision between experienced practitioners. In particular it highlights the difficulties that professionals face when they are working in specialised fields of practice that make peer support from colleagues with expert knowledge almost impossible. From their experiences they offer a three-stage model of the supervisory process that has relevance in post-qualification supervision particularly.

Chapter 4.2 is written by Lesley Rudd and Phillip Wolsey who worked together to introduce clinical supervision in a large Trust at a time of organisational change. This change took place when services for people with mental health problems and services for people with learning disabilities were being combined. This case study explores many issues faced by managers working in organisations that are part of a larger system (the NHS) and when they are working with limited resources. Despite these difficulties Rudd and Wolsey successfully introduced clinical supervision for nursing staff and for care assistants. Their account provides examples of many helpful and effective strategies as well as providing a model for clinical supervision.

The role of the supervisor is explored in Chapter 5 using data from an empirical study of professional development and nursing students' experiences of supervision. Professional development for both partners in the supervisory relationship is at the heart and soul of supervision. Through this activity practice can be explored and addressed, often providing new insights and achievement. The collaborative nature of effective supervision increases a personal sense of worth and commitment that can counterbalance the significant stress of working in health care settings. In addressing questions such as: 'How may professional development be promoted?', and 'What is effective supervision in practice?', readers can grasp from first-hand accounts what it is like to receive good supervision. From this evidence it became apparent that many mentors had difficulty understanding the requirements of their role, despite good in-service education. Other practitioners provided excellent support gained from years of experience coupled with willingness and ability to talk about their practice. These data provide a model of effective supervisory practice that has a strong empirical and theoretical basis drawn from a range of disciplines.

This leads towards the next chapter that addresses the challenge facing educators and service managers wishing to implement preparation programmes for supervisors. Chapter 6 provides an outline curriculum for such a course and explores some effective strategies for supporting supervisors. Based on professional experience as an educator, Spouse describes processes such as critical incident analysis and action learning circles as a means for busy practitioners to critically analyse and learn from their work whilst gaining increased self-confidence and competence as supervisors.

The final chapter returns to the political and social context of supervision. In addressing the question about political implications of supervision, the contributors draw upon key themes from earlier chapters and examine implications for the quality agenda and for health care providers. The chapter also explores the extent to which supervision can meet all the agendas of politicians and service providers and, indeed whether it is appropriate to expect this to be possible. This leads to further questions about the nature and intention of supervision, such as who benefits from it, and to what extent is it a bureaucratic ploy designed to cover up more profound structural deficiencies in a system that has a fundamental place in our society.

Supervision for professional development

Looking across the chapters of this book a number of themes emerge and are addressed. First is the complexity of the supervision process. It is not simply a matter of a quick chat at six-weekly intervals and a form being signed off. Supervision entails a sophisticated understanding of professional practice that is often hard to communicate. Practitioners who take on the role must be carefully selected and prepared. They must be highly competent in their field of expertise. They must be able to juggle a number of activities at one time: practice, research, management, supervision and education. They must also be able and willing to examine their practice clearly and critically. Many practitioners who are either students new to a clinical speciality or newly qualified need opportunities to work alongside an expert practitioner. In such situations their supervisor must be willing to work alongside their colleague or student and be able to guide their practice in a sensitive and educational manner.

Secondly, supervision can be dangerous to self-esteem. Being confronted by a student or a colleague who misunderstands or has different views can be a threatening experience requiring considerable maturity and sensitivity as well as peer support. For practitioners who provide supervision to colleagues working in a different setting, problems can be compounded by the limitations of their first-hand experience. As a result they have to accept their own limitations without feeling a failure and take a broader perspective. Their colleagues need generic support that fosters an ability to think and to discuss their practice honestly and critically, as well as to formulate action plans that are developmental.

Thirdly, supervision is not a cheap means of educating a workforce. Evidence suggests that effective supervision can save money by improving practice and thus reducing expensive litigation costs. But to be effective supervision takes time and cannot be introduced on a shoestring. Staff have to receive good preparation and on-going peer support. They also need to have workloads that take account of this extra responsibility and this requires more money for effective staffing and skill mix. Policies have to be supported by resources, otherwise supervision becomes an expensive paper exercise.

References

Department of Health (1989) *Working for Patients*. London, HMSO, London.
Department of Health (1991) *Medical Audit in the Hospital and the Community Health Service* HC (91) 2, January. DoH, London.
Department of Health (1993) *A Vision for the Future: the Nursing, Midwifery and Health Visiting Contribution to Health Care*. HMSO, London.
Department of Health (1998) *A First Class Service – Quality in the New NHS*. HC (91) 2, January, DoH, London.
Donabedian, A. (1966) Evaluating the quality of medical care. *Millbank Memorial Fund Quarterly* **XLIV**, no. 3, part 2, 166–205.
Ericsson, K. A., Krampe, R. Th. & Tesch-Romer, C. (1993) The role of deliberate

practice in the acquisition of expert performance. *Psychological Review* 100 (3), 363–406.

Kolb, D. A. (1984) *Experiential Learning: Experience as a Source of Learning and Development*. Prentice Hall, Englewood Cliffs.

National Committee of Inquiry into Higher Education (1997) *Higher Education in the Learning Society: Summary Report*. Chairman Sir Ron Dearing. HMSO, London.

Ovretveit, J. (1992) *Health Service Quality: An Introduction to Quality Methods in Health Services*. Blackwell Science, Oxford.

Walsh, M. & Ford, P. (1989) *Nursing Rituals: Research and Rational Actions*. Heinemann Nursing, London.

Chapter 2

Clinical Supervision – Professional Development or Management Control?

Nigel Northcott

'It never really appealed to me! The experiences of my friends left me grateful that I never had one. Reasons like "Her work's gone off the boil, we'd better do her appraisal", or "We'd better do your appraisal before you leave next week"; left me uncertain about the whole idea. I've been qualified for six years and have never actually had an appraisal. Mind you, I have done the two-day training course, but that was three years ago and it was never followed up.' *(Melanie, ward sister)*

This account was offered by one of the nurses who assisted me to complete a piece of research into appraisal for nurses (Northcott 1996) and offers immediate insight into why appraisal has not been taken up fully by nursing. Few of the nurses who contributed to my research were able to offer comprehensive and encouraging experiences of appraisal despite their appreciation of the importance and value of this form of performance feedback. Despite similar negative or non-existent experiences of appraisal the nurses all recognised the importance of getting feedback on performance, especially if it was constructive.

'Anything would be better than nothing! Mind you it wouldn't be difficult for the appraiser to be positive and encouraging; morale's so low in nursing, it would be good to feel you were appreciated.' *(Roger, D grade nurse)*

'I don't think they care! It doesn't make sense to spend so much of your resources on employing staff and not bothering to monitor how effective they are. Mind you, my only experience of having an appraisal was to be told to attend a meeting at which I was given four objectives. They were things my boss had been asked to do and she passed them on to me. Mind you she never bothered to check I'd done them and they wouldn't have done much for me! I thought appraisal was about developing people, not bossing them around. Anyway we're not doing appraisals any more; we're going to have clinical supervision instead.' (Barbara, D grade nurse)

'It's supposed to be about praise; isn't that where the word comes from? Nurses are very suspicious about appraisal, especially as management has become so macho and into controlling. If you ask me, supervision will never succeed unless nurses are convinced it's not another means to check on what they're doing.' (Chloe, nurse manager)

My research into appraisal for nurses included exploring the whole range of performance management strategies for nurses. Clinical supervision had emerged as a significant issue during the course of my work. This was to the extent that I even considered that the ideas in the third quotation above might come to pass. Clinical supervision might replace appraisal. Over a number of years the place and value of appraisal for nurses had concerned me and in early considerations of the subject I had identified the potential relationships between appraisal and nursing practice that are schematised in Fig. 2.1

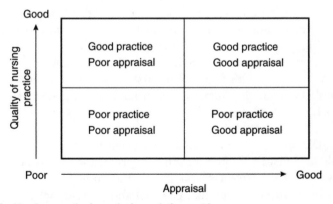

Fig. 2.1 Nursing practice/appraisal correlation matrix.

I was keen to explore what if any was the correlation between quality of nursing practice and appraisal. If this link was established I was keen to identify the characteristics of the approach to appraisal that would contribute to the development of practice and individual professionals. The grid also indicates the reverse possibility: that bad appraisal might lead to poor practice, and even that good practice could arise if appraisal was not good.

Appraisal is defined as '. . . the process of valuing the employee's worth to the organisation, with a view to increasing it' (Dutfield & Eling 1990). However, it has questionable status and uptake in nursing. A variety of settings, schemes and energies have given rise to many individual approaches to appraisal in nursing, but the lack of success of many of them is documented by the Institute of Health Service Management (1992). Their report also notes that individualised performance review (IPR) is largely confined to 'higher ranks' and is not accepted among clinical staff where the vast majority of nurses are found. The poor degree of uptake of appraisal is borne out by De la Coeur (1992) who identifies local initiatives to develop IPR but suggests that these are not widespread. The change in behaviour (learning) that can arise from appraisal can enhance the organisation and help fulfil the potential and motivation of individuals. Appraisal is, however, only one of a number of performance management strategies that may be in place in organisations.

Performance management

Performance management offers several strategies that are designed to bring about improvement and development in services to ensure an effective and efficient organisation. The strategies are designed to optimise results, increase productivity and help ensure high quality service and activity of the organisation and individuals. Within health care, performance management has the potential to inform, develop and sustain clinical practice, educational endeavours and academic achievement. During a workshop with a group of nurses I devised a diagram to help distinguish between the different performance management strategies. This has been amended a number of times since and is presented here as Fig. 2.2.

Figure 2.2 shows six performance management strategies that can be available for nurses and other health care professionals depending upon their individual assertiveness and managerial enthusiasm. All of them can contribute to organisational, personal and professional effectiveness by helping to improve the performance of the individual. To help differentiate between the six strategies, I considered how the agenda was created for each of them and Fig. 2.2 shows this as a continuum. The agenda in disciplinary action arises from line managers; the agenda for clinical supervision from the practitioner and that for appraisal are a joint responsibility. It is feasible that the professionally astute individual would report their own shortcomings to management and submit them-

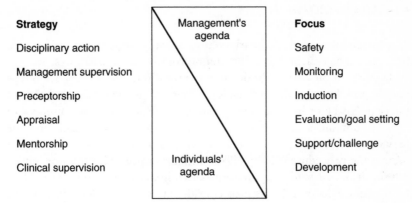

Strategy		Focus
	Management's agenda	
Disciplinary action		Safety
Management supervision		Monitoring
Preceptorship		Induction
Appraisal		Evaluation/goal setting
Mentorship		Support/challenge
Clinical supervision	Individuals' agenda	Development

Fig. 2.2

selves to professional adjudication with regard to disciplinary action and management supervision, but this cannot be expected. Such self-submission is only likely to occur in an organisation that is truly developmental.

Uncertainty about the definitions of these terms is indicated in the literature, and Morton-Cooper and Palmer (1993) offer a simple glossary in a preface to their book on mentorship. Butterworth *et al.* (1996) identify the difficulty in distinguishing between clinical supervision, preceptorship and individual performance review (appraisal), and a definition quagmire is reported with regard to the role of mentor (Hagerty 1986). Much confusion exists between preceptorship and mentoring (Brennan 1993), and mentorship is identified elsewhere as a 'slippery concept' (Cross 1986). Eddison (1994), in commenting that all nurses should have someone to turn to, suggests the title is unimportant. Exactly what can be expected of and what is intended by 'someone whom nurses can turn to' is unfortunately bound up in this confusion about the different roles and strategies. This chapter explores the six performance management strategies that operate for nurses, alongside three organisation dimensions that will significantly influence the process: organisational culture, the psychological contract and motivational theories.

The six performance management strategies

We will now look at six performance management strategies, namely, disciplinary action, management supervision, preceptorship, mentorship, clinical supervision, and appraisal.

Disciplinary Action

The procedure in disciplinary action usually follows an agreement between management and trade union/professional body representatives and focuses upon safety. The decision to take disciplinary action should be based upon the belief that a nurse's performance is such that patient/client safety might be or has been compromised. The strategy has a number of possible outcomes depending upon the severity of the breach and the previous performance of the individual. If a serious breach of conduct occurs, the procedure usually allows for suspension from duty or indeed instant dismissal from employment. Disciplinary action should be taken when failure in performance is considered to be reckless, illegal (for example theft or assault) or unprofessional (for example breach of confidence or accepting favours). If the disciplinary action is taken as a result of a serious breach of professional conduct, this may also trigger a report being made to the professional statutory body who will decide upon the action it should take.

Management supervision

Management supervision is the continuous responsibility of all nurses in management positions, and focuses primarily on monitoring the performance of staff. The strategy involves drawing to the attention of the individual unacceptable or questionable practice against agreed standards, policies and protocols. This should be done in privacy and as soon after the incident as is possible. Failure to respond to this feedback can lead to formal disciplinary action as indicated above. Management supervision should address unsatisfactory performance that is not reckless, for example a drug error that results from human error, or errors of judgement that do not significantly compromise safety. Appropriate use and operation of management supervision can also help eliminate the need for disciplinary action by addressing shortcomings in practice before they become a threat to patient care. Management supervision is designed and intended to improve performance and not to punish staff. The agenda for management supervision is identified by the manager, and the individual nurse is unlikely to be able to choose who this will be. Clarification about how management supervision operates in a particular post can be sought by a nurse from a more senior colleague or from the personnel department.

It might also be useful at this point to note that the term 'management supervision' is derived from the word 'supervise' and implies watching over, checking and correcting. However, once again development should

govern the activity. If management supervision is done disc‌
private), immediately or as soon as possible and constructively, it‌
means to the development of practice and individuals. Regrettably a
controlling attitude often dominates that may lead to demoralisation and
no chance of learning from the error.

Preceptorship

Preceptorship was identified in the *Post-Registration and Practice Report*
from the United Kingdom Central Council (1990) as good practice,
especially for newly qualified nurses and those newly appointed to a post.
The role focuses upon the induction of newly appointed staff, with the
preceptor operating in an educational capacity to provide a role model
and resource (Chickerella & Lutz 1981). In this relationship, the agenda is
created by the members of staff, with the preceptor offering useful insight
into the new role, and the individual free to ask questions. The preceptor is
likely to be appointed, in which case they should be chosen for their
organisational knowledge and interpersonal skills as well as professional
expertise. The period of engagement will depend upon need and is likely to
taper off as the new member of staff gains confidence, and indeed may
lead to the establishment of clinical supervision.

Mentorship

Mentorship is the process of helping another to learn and enhance their
professional role (Watkins & Whalley 1993). A mentor should be
someone you trust (Acton Ray *et al.* 1992; Spouse 1996) and, like Obi
Wan Kanobi in the Star Wars Trilogy, someone you can turn to when in
difficulty! This person may be relevant as a career advisor following
qualification or as required by the United Kingdom Central Council for
Nurses, Midwives and Health Visitors to be someone identified for each
pre-registration student. The focus of mentorship is clearly one where
support and challenge should be offered equally to ensure professional
growth and vision. To avoid the pitfalls of a 'toxic' mentor (Darling
1985), the choice of mentor should preferably remain with the individual.
This may not always be possible if time working in the specific location
and the duration of the relationship is going to be short. If possible the
choices should include the person, the purpose and the time span of the
relationship. This approach requires the organisation to identify possible
mentors and to provide them with training and support. However, it must
be recognised that mentors may be sought from outside the organisation,
and the use of a model in which the mentor is appointed may be more
aligned to management supervision or preceptorship.

Clinical supervision

Clinical supervision entered the professional language of nursing in the early 1990s with a flurry of interest, uncertainty and suspicion, in part I believe as a result of nurses' experience of appraisal. Was clinical supervision yet another attempt to control nurses, as one of my respondents had suggested? The term 'supervision' had long been associated with psychologists (Hogan 1964), midwives (UKCC 1993) and managers in general, but this has created an uncertain heritage. It was clearly identified within psychology as a developmental strategy. Stoltenberg & Delworth (1987) identify four stages of supervisee development. These stages indicate how the process can advance a practitioner from a state of dependency, through explorer to competence and eventually on to mastery. Midwifery supervision, however, was established in such a way that it is tied into and compromised by the administrative structure (Curtiss 1992). There are criticisms that it is punitive, inflexible and confused by its managerial associations (Chaffer 1998). Walker (1988) argues for a supervisor who is a respected clinical peer who can assist in professional development and not operate as an agent of line management. Isherwood (1988) is similarly unequivocal in suggesting that midwifery supervision should be divorced from management control. It is against this background that a national drive to establish clinical supervision for nurses was undertaken (Bishop 1994).

Clinical supervision is the latest performance management strategy to be identified as significant in the repertoire. A universally accepted definition of clinical supervision has yet to emerge, and indeed even the term has been questioned. Clinical supervision shares with all the performance management strategies the intention of developing practice. The concept may be better appreciated if the word is broken down as 'clinical supervision', which focuses the term on to a visionary role. There are three aims of clinical supervision that are mutually inclusive: managerial insight, support, and education (Kadushin 1976; Procter 1986), which clearly suggest it is a developmental tool.

Figure 2.2 clearly indicates that clinical supervision is a performance management strategy in which the agenda is driven by the individual nurse. This agenda, arising from their practice, uses reflection and critical incident analysis to help sustain and develop practice. It is important to acknowledge that the managerial component is not one created as an aspect of a hierarchy or as a means of control but as a collegial action to safeguard standards. Indeed the process is dependent upon the individual nurse creating the agenda, and unless the climate is conducive to this the nurse may either be untruthful or decline to participate. Clinical supervision can only operate as a voluntary activity and therefore management must make it attractive; it must offer it in a distinctly developmental manner.

Appraisal

Appraisal should, as indicated in Fig. 2.2, operate as a mutual process where there is joint responsibility to evaluate performance and negotiate goals or learning contracts for the forthcoming period. However, there is no apparent consensus about the term 'appraisal' in the literature. Dutfield & Eling (1990) state that studies by the Institute of Personnel Management suggest 82% of UK companies operate some form of performance review scheme (appraisal). Deming, cited in Peters (1987), suggests that it takes the average employee six months to recover from an appraisal. I would question whether this is a result of the appraisal or of the way that it is conducted.

Three vital aspects of appraisal will need to be addressed if success is to be achieved and these are:

- Purpose of appraisal
- Agreement
- Commitment

Purpose of appraisal

The purpose of appraisal is an echo of the literature on the value of evaluation (Macintosh & Frith 1984) in that appraisals may:

- Help assess training needs
- Improve current performance
- Set objectives for the future
- Assist in planning decisions, and in reviewing achievements and recent performance
- Assist in selection and in the development of potential

All are aspects that might be seen as of value to both sides, if indeed 'sides' is the correct term. However, there are two quite challenging purposes for appraisal, weeding out and assessing value, which are alluded to by Burgess (1989). I strongly contend that appraisal should not be the sole factor for either or both of these, but it might play some small part. Personally I feel the central purpose should be to develop the workforce resource. If it is to be linked to 'weeding out', or, for example performance-related pay, these must be clearly stated at the outset, with formally agreed criteria, but with cognisance of the impact that this may have upon the whole process.

I would contend that weeding out should be the remit of disciplinary action and then only if the member of staff demonstrates reckless action. Appraisal should be left to reflect its possible etymological origin of praise.

Agreement

Before an appraisal scheme is introduced, clear negotiation is needed to generate an acceptable scheme. In my own experience, individual performance review (IPR) in the National Health Service (NHSTA 1986) was presented as a management *fait accompli* and subsequently saw limited success. In my current role I am engaged in a number of centres assisting with the introduction of clinical supervision and fear the same problems may happen to it if a too prescriptive approach is used.

Appraisal and clinical supervision should be introduced as collaborative ventures between staff and managers, recognising the developmental benefit they can have for individual and organisational productivity.

Commitment

Without commitment no scheme of appraisal will succeed. A scheme with purposes agreed by all involved has great potential, whereas the imposed scheme with covert and/or openly negative (management control) purposes is liable both to failure and to meet the types of difficulties often associated with appraisal.

These three areas are not sequential as may be suggested here. They interact with each other, and in their absence it is unlikely that a scheme of appraisal will succeed. Indeed I contend failure to address them has been one reason why appraisal schemes often become bureaucratic nightmares.

Burgess (1989) reinforces this notion with three valuable attributes to good appraisal schemes. They should be:

- Non-hierarchical – a collegial developmental activity
- Non-judgemental – based upon criteria not opinions
- Research-based – underpinned by evidence

This supports the idea that appraisal is a tool for staff development which has consequential management benefit and by which groups of staff may collectively agree performance criteria and evaluation strategies rather than have them imposed by managerial decree.

From my own research (Northcott 1996) I identified eight reflections about appraisal that offer insight into how it might be implemented successfully. The eight reflections are:

(1) Appraisal informs and helps guide the professional fulfilment of nurses
(2) The central focus of appraisal should be development
(3) Preparation for undertaking appraisal requires particular education and training
(4) Appraisal is an investment in the nursing staff
(5) Appraisal is a significant strategy in personnel management
(6) Suspicion and indifference are features of the current culture of appraisal
(7) The evidence and records of appraisal will significantly influence effectiveness
(8) Appraisal should reflect the ethos of holism

(1) Appraisal informs and helps guide the professional fulfilment of nurses

The formal contract of employment that a nurse holds is only one of the obligations to practise and perform well. The psychological contract (Mullins 1996) of mutual expectation between a nurse and their employer is an important component of the nurse's work. Appraisal is one of the ways that the nurse's formal contract can be developed, by providing feedback and evaluation of performance, but the exact way this is done should reflect the psychological contract. Appraisal has the potential to help overcome the doubts and concerns about the quality of care delivered that individual practitioners can only partially obtain for themselves. The assertion that good appraisal could ensure good performance was confirmed by my research by the nurses, with acknowledgement that good performance may also arise when appraisal is bad! However, it was recognised that performance in the latter case could be further enhanced if the appraisal had been good.

(2) The central focus of appraisal should be development

The moral commitment and psychological contract that are central to nursing contain within them the importance of care: to be a good nurse. It is for this reason that appraisal should operate as a developmental activity to affirm the natural intention of nurses to strive to improve and to extend their skills. Areas for development should be negotiated within a supportive professional dialogue that recognises the natural need and desire of each nurse to develop.

It was evident from my research that the use of appraisal to control nurses was a strong reason for the degree of alienation associated with it. Control as the overt or covert intention of appraisal is unlikely to be wholly successful and is likely to inhibit the developmental growth of nurses. The fundamental contradiction of the two purposes, i.e. control and development, indicates that they are mutually exclusive. They must be separated in the organisation's performance management strategies. The need to control and manage inadequate or inappropriate performance is a legitimate activity but one that is distinctly separate from appraisal. Equally the use of appraisal as a comparative/normative exercise was rejected by the nurses in favour of an approach that strives for professional development. The sterile cascading of objectives down the organisation was reported to feel more like attempts to control the nurses. Negotiation of mutually agreed objectives would help the empowerment of nurses who might then be better placed to empower patients.

(3) Preparation for undertaking appraisal requires particular education and training.
The establishment of elaborate and complex education and training events was felt to be time consuming, as bottlenecks arose as nurses waited to attend these events. This had generated delays in the introduction of appraisal to nurses. The use of local guidelines rather than prescriptive methods for undertaking appraisal would allow for locally based cascades which could be adapted to the exact needs of the staff. It was evident from my research that learning by doing had been a successful way of implementing appraisal and, if this is underpinned by clear guidelines and support from colleagues, it could be the basis for an effective scheme.

(4) Appraisal is an investment in the nursing staff
The acknowledgement and demonstration of appraisal as an investment strategy requires a commitment of time and other resources that would reap benefits for the organisation. The returns from this investment might include improved performance and motivation of the staff, as well as improvements in staff retention, quality of care and productivity.

(5) Appraisal is a significant strategy in personnel management
The value and importance of appraisal as a personnel management strategy to enrich and enhance the performance and well-being of nursing staff were identified by Northcott (1996). In this study appraisal was acknowledged as an important strategy in the development and enrichment of nurses, despite the anxiety that it had generated for them in the past. Performance development was recognised as a lifelong process by nurses in my study. It was acknowledged that some degree of monitoring ('policing') of nursing practice is required to underpin accountability, but not in order to punish shortcomings. It was emphasised that any such monitoring should be intended to develop and not to control nurses. The feeling of being taken for granted and of not being given encouragement had been significant factors in the growth of job dissatisfaction. The

absence of regular systematic praise and feedback could not be compensated for by occasional comments about good performance, or by appraisal that is triggered by failings in performance.

(6) Suspicion and indifference are features of the current culture of appraisal

Experiences of appraisal have generated an appraisal culture in nursing that leaves it hampered by suspicion and apathy. A considerable degree of indifference exists among many of the nurses who are responsible for conducting as well as for receiving appraisal. This arises for a number of reasons that include nurses' previous poor experiences, uncertainty about the value of appraisal, and the failure of management to recognise the long-term investment that it offers. Nurses who celebrated appraisal were those for whom it was a developmental activity or those who have appraisal linked to their performance-related pay, the latter group for obvious if not very different reasons.

(7) The evidence and records of appraisal will significantly influence effectiveness

To overcome the concerns about confidentiality and access to appraisal evidence the research confirmed that records should be held by the individual nurse and seen as their property. This would reinforce the primary intention of appraisal as a developmental activity, and precludes the use of these records for other purposes without the nurse's consent. The evidence could contribute to the departmental evaluation, or be used in support of career enhancement, but only if advanced by the nurse. This approach accommodates the proposals from the UKCC (1990) that require individual nurses to create a personal professional profile. The profile should contain evidence of competence and of development; this is the ideal location to store appraisal evidence. Adoption of nurse-held records also overcomes the bureaucratic problems of how long to keep the records, who should have legitimate access to them, and whose responsibility they are.

(8) Appraisal should reflect the ethos of holism

Appraisal had limited impact for nurses in my study. This was in part as a result of the failure to acknowledge the importance of holism that encompasses nursing practice. Appraisal schemes were operated without taking account of the contradiction they presented to the caring nurse if an apathetic, hasty and punitive approach to appraisal was used. This presents a picture that is the antithesis of the quality care the profession strives to achieve. Appraisal needs to operate in a culture where critique is valued and to be established within a relationship where challenges to practice are met by the genuine intention to provide support.

Professional development or management control?

What is clearly common to all the performance management strategies is the intention that underpins the process: development or control? This will be significantly informed by the organisational culture and the psychological contract along with the views of motivation attributed to the staff. These three dimensions will impact upon the whole organisation with regard to appraisal and its associated performance management strategies, and cannot be overlooked. My own research confirmed that suspicion and indifference are features of the current culture of appraisal. Given that nurses have the responsibility to evaluate their performance and to consider ways of developing their practice established within their Code of Conduct, they should recognise and receive the challenge and ongoing support of appraisal with their manager as a way to help achieve this. It has been reported that performance appraisal in the NHS is 'littered with valiant attempts that have died a fairly early death' (Gourlay 1986). This is a situation that might have been remedied if the underlying philosophy had not been one of management control. Had mutual responsibility with multiple evidence evaluation, negotiated goals/contracts and ongoing support been features of a developmental approach, the situation might have been very different. Fitzgerald (1989, p.95) suggests that appraisal is seen by nurses to be of little value: indeed some have suggested that it is time wasting, punitive and sometimes destructive. These doubts and experiences I believe have infected our view and expectation of clinical supervision and arise primarily because appraisal is operated as a form of managerial control. Clinical supervision has been established for almost a decade within the nursing literature. However, I very much doubt that more than 30% of nurses receive it. This situation arises partly because, like appraisal, the practitioners themselves do not push for it, which is no surprise if management control dominates the process. There are of course many approaches to appraisal and clinical supervision, and not all of them are victim to the difficulties raised here.

Culture, the psychological contract and theories of motivation

Appraisal, clinical supervision and the associated performance management strategies do not operate in a vacuum. The environment within which they operate is created by the psychological contract, culture and motivational views of the organisation. Positive links have been established between a constructive culture and morale, staff retention, service enhancement and even decreased mortality of patients (McDaniel & Stumpf 1993).

The Culture

'... how things are done around here' *(Egan 1994)*

Culture will have a powerful impact upon appraisal and clinical supervision. Hawkins & Shohet (1989 a, b) emphasise the impact of culture on performance management and they identify five different and distinct types:

- Personal pathology
- The bureaucratic culture
- Watch your back
- Reactive/crisis driven
- Learning/developmental

Personal pathology

This culture speaks for itself: it sees the staff as the agents of mistakes and failings and seeks out who to blame. This more often than not leads to a punitive attitude to correct performance.

The bureaucratic culture

The clearly laid down rules, regulations and lists of procedures of a bureaucracy inhibit the performance of professionals by prescribing how and when work should be undertaken. This can strip patients of their individuality, undermine the ability and potential of professionals and create a cumbersome and unresponsive organisation. Menzies (1960) was one of the early nurses to identify the depersonalised nature of a bureaucracy and was critical of the breakdown of the work to be done into tasks with little regard for the people involved. Within this culture, performance management is established within a set of rules rather than reasons and creates a sense of control rather than development.

Watch-your-back culture

This functions by 'showing up' other departments or individuals who are failing, in an arena of competition. It is a culture where sharpening the competitive edge, rather than genuinely and broadly ensuring development, exists and is one in which elitism arises.

Reactive crisis culture

This is a problem-solving culture where attention is focused only on immediate problems with no concern for development or visionary activities. This culture operates in many busy departments especially if the leadership is short-sighted and tentative. It more often wheels in performance management strategies in response to failings rather than seeing problems as part of ongoing development.

The learning/development culture

This culture best illustrates the developmental organisation and is one where growth, development and learning are all central. The notion of the 'learning company' (Pedlar *et al.* 1991) is a clear example of this culture, where the following exist:

- Learning is seen as a lifelong activity for all staff
- All work situations may potentially create learning opportunities
- Problems are learning opportunities
- Good practices arise from exploring learning cycles
- Feedback exists at all levels and is on-going
- Time is an expected dimension of change
- Regular review and evaluation are part of the individual and organisational activity

Performance management is an essential tool of the developmental culture and is a proactive strategy for developing the staff and the organisation collaboratively.

The psychological contract

The mutual expectations between the individual and the organisation have an important impact on behaviour, but do not form part of the formal contract of employment. Within this psychological contract (Mullins 1996) the nurse should be able to expect: a safe workplace, to be treated with respect as an individual, to be given opportunities for self-enhancement and to be supported and challenged to develop their potential. The organisation might expect: loyalty, a diligent approach to work, acceptance of the ideology and striving to sustain the image of the organisation in exchange. The significance of the psychological contract to both appraisal and clinical supervision is that it helps establish the culture within which a philosophy of control or development will be located.

Motivational theories

Within the field of motivational psychology two particular concepts help shed light on the perspective of development or control as a means to motivate and manage performance (Herzberg 1959; McGregor 1960). McGregor put forward two suppositions about human nature and behaviour at work, Theory X and Theory Y.

Theory X represents the assumptions of organisations considered to be traditional and based on power and thus hierarchy. To maintain such positions, concepts of the worker undermine any worth that s/he may have. These assumptions depend upon images of workers as lacking ambition, avoiding responsibility, lazy, disliking work, and in need of direction/coercion, control and the threat of punishment if management objectives are to be met.

By contrast Theory Y represents more enlightened and humanitarian approaches. These regard people as self-directing, and highly motivated to find purpose from life when valued and respected. Such beliefs represent assumptions of current research knowledge and celebrate the integration of both individual and organisational goals. The McGregor X assumption implies the need to coerce staff to perform, in a personal pathology culture where sanctions, coercion and control dominate. This culture seeks to find scapegoats and attributes blame to individuals. It uses financial rewards to motivate staff and would, worst of all, assume that the nurses do not really want to care for patients! Assumption Y adopts a far more positive attitude towards staff and would commend developmental approaches to performance management given the staff's intrinsic commitment and intentions. Herzberg's two-factor theory (Herzberg 1959) provides a strategy to manage such approaches. He identifies 'hygiene factors' that serve to prevent dissatisfaction and 'motivational factors' that offer satisfaction. Herzberg stresses again the benefit of positive encouragement to promote performance from both sets of factors. Over time these theories have been the subject of criticism and re-examination but the premise that reinforcing good behaviour is more successful than punishing the unacceptable remains firmly established.

Conclusions

To ensure appraisal may be perceived and operated as a developmental tool, attitudes must reflect beliefs about the workforce based upon respecting and valuing each member of the workforce. This affords each member equal rights and the ability to make a contribution which can be enhanced through continuing professional development. Congruent with such beliefs a number of factors will need to be clearly established which depend upon commitment. These factors are enshrined within codes of professional conduct and standards of practice when concerned with clients and patients. Unless they are also enshrined within management structures and interpersonal relationships, such codes of practice are worthless. As with client/patient interactions, staff must also be provided with uninterrupted contact time to ensure a comprehensive assessment to precede a development plan which describes the behaviours expected in the role. This should include a job description and performance standards that are clear and understandable to both the member of staff and the manager and have been agreed well in advance of any performance review. Unless such documents are available, what criteria can be used to appraise the practitioner or how will s/he or indeed anyone else be able to judge performance or learning needs? Development can then be planned in the light of best practice and evidence of what is achievable that can be obtained from a variety of (literature) sources. The appraisal of performance should be a reflection of overall performance rather than based upon single incidents of good or bad performance. Single episodes may be used as critical incidents for discussion, analysis and managing (Brookfield 1987) within supervision. Records of the outcome of such discussions may be used during performance review meetings. They provide a resource that gives a variety of perspectives on individual performance (triangulation from a number of sources). Critical incidents should never be used as the sole content of appraisal and should not bias overall performance evaluation. Beliefs about quality enhancement use mistakes as opportunities for development and learning, not only by the worker but also by the manager. Mistakes are often associated with poor resources, insufficient training or inadequate policies (Berwick 1989), and practitioners should not be used as scapegoats for structural or organisational problems. Copies of all the records of the events must be kept both by the appraisee and by the appraiser. A progressive, trusting organisation would leave all record-keeping responsibilities with the individual practitioner. These should include agreement of key areas for development, the action plan and where further support may need to be offered. Performance development should not be a one-off activity but should be on-going with regular contact to ensure support is available and development is proceeding.

These conclusions are essentially derived from work on appraisal, but are equally applicable to clinical supervision. If these two performance management strategies are both intended as developmental tools, then the same principles apply. The differences relate to timescale. Appraisal has an annual evaluative phase and an annual goal/objective phase. Clinical supervision has a more day-to-day feel to it: it is a dynamic tool for analysing and learning from everyday practice issues. These two processes can thereby be readily linked together, clinical supervision contributing to the review and goal setting as well as being an opportunity to revisit goals during the year. I would compound this relationship by suggesting that the same colleague could be both appraiser and clinical supervisor if the nurse agreed and if the process was truly a developmental one. The difference may be that the nurse is predominantly responsible for setting the agenda in clinical supervision and the appraiser for leading the negotiation in appraisal.

These issues and this chapter make no attempt to recommend systems for use. However, given the current demands for effective and efficient practice expectation as well as the professional demands of lifelong learning and periodic re-registration, they are both unavoidable as well as highly desirable. I am advocating that appraisal and clinical supervision become fully integrated parts of the professional portfolio, providing useful evidence for the individual, particularly of personal practice development.

In the true spirit of bottom-up approaches to management (Handy 1976), schemes of appraisal and clinical supervision are dependent upon the context in which they will operate and therefore they should be developed with the specific staff group in mind, not as a national, organisational or departmental initiative. For example, Handy (1990) suggests reformulating appraisals as self-development contracts, to correct in part the common assumption that appraisals are judgement, not help. This also reinforces the focus on individuals and their needs and not directly the organisation's needs. However, by assisting the staff to recognise good work and function both effectively and efficiently, the organisation will benefit. This is in contrast to schemes in which objectives are passed down hierarchies by layers of management and individual ownership is minimal. Appraisal and clinical supervision should not be designed by management and imposed upon the staff, but facilitated by means of organisational guidelines that are drawn up collaboratively and applied flexibly. There are many ways to provide clinical supervision and appraisal and the organisation with developmental intentions recognises this and seeks to synergise with the staff to effect the best outcomes.

References

Acton Ray *et al.* (1992) *Mentoring: A Core-skills Pack*. Crewe and Alsager College.
Berwick, D. M. (1989) Continuous improvement as an ideal in health care. *New England Journal of Medicine* **321**(1), 53–56.
Bishop, V. (1994) Clinical supervision for an accountable profession. *Nursing Times* **90** (39), 35–7.
Brennan, A. (1993) Preceptorship: is it a workable concept? *Nursing Standard* **7** (52), 34–36.

Brookfield, S. (1987) *Developing Critical Thinkers*. Open University Press, Milton Keynes.

Burgess, R. (1989) *Rethinking Appraisal and Assessment*. Open University Press, Milton Keynes.

Butterworth, T., Bishop, V., Carson, J., & White E. (1996) *The NHS Triple Project: An Exploration of a Methodology by which Clinical Supervision in Nursing can be Evaluated* (On-going research) Manchester University, Manchester.

Chaffer, D. (1998) The midwifery model of supervision. *Nursing Times Learning Curve* 2 (6), 5 August.

Chickerella, B & Lutz, W. (1981) Professional nurturing: preceptorship for undergraduate nursing students. *American Journal of Nursing* 81 (1), 107–9.

Cross, K. P. (1986) Forward. In *Effective Teaching and Mentoring* (L.A. Daloz, ed.), Jossey Bass, San Francisco.

Curtiss, P. (1992) Supervision in clinical midwifery practice. In *Clinical Supervision and Mentorship Nursing* (A. Butterworth & J. Faugier, eds). Chapman & Hall, London.

Darling, L. (1985) What to do about toxic mentors. *Journal of Nursing Administration* 15 (5), 43–4.

De la Coeur, J. (1992) Assessment of staff appraisal systems. *British Journal of Nursing* 1 (2), 99–102.

Dutfield, M. & Eling, C. (1990) *The Communicating Manager* Element Books, Shaftesbury.

Eddison, G. (1994) Monitoring mentoring. *Nursing Standard* 8 (30) 99.

Egan, G. (1994) Cultivate your culture. *Management Today* April, 38–42.

Fitzgerald, M. (1989) Performance planning and review. In *Managing Nursing Work* (B. Vaughan & M. Pilmoor, eds), Scutari Press, London.

Gourlay, R. (1986) Performance appraisal, a systematic approach. *Health Care Management* 1 (1), 32–5.

Hagerty, B. (1986) A second look at mentors. *Nursing Outlook* 34 (1), 16–19.

Handy, C. (1976) *Understanding Organisations*. Penguin, London.

Handy, C. (1990) *The Age of Unreason*. Arrow, London.

Hawkins, P. & Shohet, R. (1989a) *Rethinking Appraisal and Assessment*. Open University Press, Milton Keynes.

Hawkins, P. & Shohet, R. (1989b) *Supervision in the Helping Professions*. Open University Press, Milton Keynes.

Herzberg, F. (1959) *The Motivation to Work*. John Wiley, New York.

Hogan, R. (1964) Issues and approaches in supervision. *Psychotherapy Theory, Research and Practice* 1, 139–41.

Institute of Health Service Management (1992) *Performance Related Pay and United Kingdom Nursing* No. 235. IHSM, University of Sussex.

Isherwood, K. (1988) Friend or watchdog? *Nursing Times* 84 (24), 65.

Kadushin, A. (1976) *Supervision in Social Work*. Columbia University Press, New York.

Macintosh, H. & Frith, D. (1984) *A Teacher's Guide to Assessment*. Stanley Thornes, Cheltenham.

McDaniel, C. & Stumpf, L. (1993) The organisational culture. *Journal of Nursing Administration* 4, 54–60.

McGregor, D. (1960) *The Human Side of Enterprise*. McGraw Hill, New York.

Menzies, I. (1960) The functioning of social systems as a defence against anxiety. Tavistock Pamphlet No. 3. Tavistock Institute of Human Relations, London.

Morton-Cooper, A. & Palmer, A. (1993) *Mentoring and Preceptorship*. Blackwell Science, Oxford.

Mullins, L. (1996) *Management and Organisational Behaviour*, 4th edn. Pitman, London.

National Health Service Training Authority (1986) *Individualised Performance Review*. NHSTA, Bristol.

Northcott, N. (1996) Appraisal and professional fulfilment of nursing staff in Oxfordshire. Unpublished PhD thesis, University of Southampton.

Pedlar, M., Burgoyne, J. & Boydell, T. (1991) *The Learning Company*. McGraw Hill, New York.

Peters, T. (1987) *Thriving on Chaos*. Pan, London.

Procter, B. (1986) Supervision: A co-operative exercise in accountability. In *Enabling and Ensuring* (M. Marken. & M. Payne, eds), Leicestershire National Youth Bureau and Council for Education and Training in Youth and Community Work.

Spouse, J. (1996) The effective mentor: A model for student-centred learning in clinical practice. *Nursing Times Research* 1 (2), 120–33.

Stoltenberg, C. & Delworth, U. (1987) *Supervising Counsellors and Therapists*. Jossey Bass, San Francisco.

United Kingdom Central Council for Nursing, Midwifery and Health Visiting (UKCC) (1990) *The Post-Registration Education and Practice Project*. UKCC, London.

United Kingdom Central Council for Nursing, Midwifery and Health Visiting (UKCC) (1992) *Code of Professional Conduct*. UKCC, London.

United Kingdom Central Council for Nursing, Midwifery and Health Visiting (1993) *Midwives' Rules*. UKCC, London.

Walker, M. (1988) Scared to be midwives? *Association of Radical Midwives Magazine* September, 13–14.

Watkins, C. & Whalley, C. (1993) *Mentoring: Resources for School Based Development*. Harlow, Longman.

Chapter 3
Personal Accounts of Supervision

Introduction

Readers working as supervisors may well recognise many of the problematic situations described here. Those who have had little experience of supervision can perhaps take comfort that they may encounter the same difficulties described by the writers but feel heartened to know how common such experiences are. We hope you will recognise that learning to supervise others is a complex process that takes time and practice to become proficient and that this book will provide some support during the challenges.

Organising the sequence of the critical incidents was difficult because of their individual nature. In the end we decided to start with Barbara Lovelady's classical dilemma of teaching technical skills to a new member of staff which are not maintained due to insufficient supervision from colleagues. Her critical incident encompasses the complexity of what at first may appear to be a simple task but which if conducted incorrectly can lead to disaster. It also communicates what Ericsson and his colleagues identified as the necessity for repetitive supervised practice (Ericsson *et al.*, 1993). This supervision must be effective for all levels of staff and at all times. Her account illustrates how difficult it is to achieve when working in busy clinical settings or under staffing constraints. The second contribution is from an experienced mental health nurse working in an acute care setting in a general hospital. Dave Roberts provides an example of expert practice where he is able to reflect-in-action about his interactions with his client. His narrative gives us insight into what this term can mean and how we can learn to use it, especially when facing difficult dilemmas. Lorna Cowan's contribution provides a startling and forceful account of the difficulties of supervising whilst being mindful of the needs of her clients in the community setting. Her critical incident illuminates the complexity of the supervisory process and the number of factors that have to be taken into account. The uncertain environment of health care practice where clients and practitioners can face danger at any moment requires constant vigilance by the senior practitioner. The interactional nature of health care practice means the supervisor has to be thinking about three people (at least) at any one time. This links well with Barbara's problem of staff having insufficient time or perhaps awareness to consider the needs of the new staff member. In Lorna's example she is working with a pre-registration midwifery student and her insights arising from the experience provide a sound basis for any practitioner to consider when supervising others. They make a fitting introduction to the subsequent narratives that begin to unpick some of the issues that she raises.

Charlotte Chesson explores an aspect of her experiences of supervising a colleague when working as team leader in an acute medical nursing unit. Her epilogue reflections identify the importance of establishing a supportive relationship with her colleague, and she then provides some insights as to how this can be created. Concepts of support are developed further by Mary Kavanagh who narrates her experiences of working with an occupational therapy student in a mental health setting. She identifies how a student's personal history can influence the triangular relationship between supervisor and patient and its subsequent impact on the nature of professional practice. One aspect of Mary's narrative that is almost taken for granted by most writers is the importance of regular and frequent meetings between supervisor and supervisee. This is particularly important in situations in which a strong relationship has not already been established. In the following chapter (4.2), Janet Gregson is supervised by a colleague whom she had known for several years and with whom she had negotiated their supervisory sessions on the basis of this relationship. This is not always possible, particularly when supervising students or colleagues without the opportunity to establish a good working relationship beforehand. Mary identifies that her student spent half of her placement 'shadowing her'. This provided an opportunity for them get to know each other and to develop a trusting working relationship. Such a relationship is stressed by all the contributors as being important and permiting learning to take place through challenging existing (mis)-conceptions. Such observations probably have as great relevance for all practitioners and not just students.

The sixth case study describes one supervisor's response to a student who is having difficulty with his interpersonal relationships. Krysia Lewandowski describes the very great risk that she took to confront her male radiography student Sam, and how it successfully enabled him to grow both personally and professionally. In her narrative she explores the familiar environment in which many practitioners prefer to isolate colleagues unable to relate effectively, rather than to find ways of helping them to learn the necessary skills. Such practices are common throughout our society and are well documented in many performance reviews. Having developed a supportive relationship with Sam she is able to understand the origin of his problems. By her willingness to challenge him Krysia breaks the trap and frees Sam to reach his potential. In her evaluation of the experience, Krysia uses Taylor's model of the learning process sequence to explore what took place for Sam. In doing so she describes the difficulties encountered by many adults returning to education (Taylor 1987). By contrast, and towards the end of a professional programme, Claire Louise Hatton describes her dilemma when supervising a senior acupuncture student. She was conscious that he was not practising in a manner that encompassed the values and beliefs of their discipline and sought ways to communicate this perception. Her narrative provides a vivid description of the essence of professional practice that may sometimes be overlooked in competency-driven assessment frameworks and which is often hard to describe. A narrative of supporting transition through a learning process experience is written by Louise Dumas who works in a French Canadian School of Nursing. She describes a critical incident that has a spiral nature. Louise is giving distant support to a colleague who is a clinical supervisor (clinical teacher). The clinical supervisor is working with an experienced colleague who has returned to full-time education. The post-registration student has now gone back to work in her own ward and is experiencing difficulties. Using the Dumas tool she illustrates a process that this conscientious and caring supervisor used to support her student and which Louise subsequently used to support her. Louise's account illustrates the stages through which many people travel when encountering new ways of thinking and acting. She also argues that, by using a structured framework, practitioners can develop their practice through discussion or journal keeping.

The concluding examples of supervised practice are given by two recent students, Sally Ballard and Lisa Benrud-Larson. They provide accounts of exemplary practice that both supported and challenged their professional development in very different contexts. Sally writes as a final year nursing student working on a unit for older persons in the UK and Lisa was learning to become a clinical psychologist in the United States. They both describe experiences of working with exemplary supervisors who were confident in their own professional practice and who were willing to draw out their students' knowledge rather than to impose their own. Fundamental to both these experiences was the nature of the relationship they had been able to develop with their supervisors and the time that they could use to explore their practice. As a result of these key processes to successful supervision, Lisa and Sally gained confidence to develop their own problem-solving skills as well as to acknowledge their limitations and to seek help. These narratives provide a fitting conclusion to the chapter, giving hope and reassurance that whilst the supervisory role is complex and challenging, even painful sometimes for all who are involved, it can be enormously rewarding and effective. In addition everyone involved moved closer to developing their skills of learning throughout their lifetime.

Writing critical incidents of supervision

It may be of interest to some readers to know how this collection of personal accounts and reflections was developed. In many respects the critical incidents provide data for a qualitative research activity. The writers were all given the same information and were asked to make the same essential contribution. Twelve clinicians representing a range of orthodox and complimentary health and social welfare professions were invited to make a contribution to the book. Following tentative enquiries about their willingness to make a contribution we held a meeting for them to meet each other and to discuss any concerns that they may have had. They had already received a copy of the book proposal that outlined the content of each chapter and a paper describing the nature of critical incident analysis. They were also provided with examples of frameworks for analysing a critical incident and some information about participating in an action learning cycle. We had anticipated that contributors may have wished to use this meeting to think through what they would write about. Although several had not met each other before and may have felt uncomfortable about exposing their concerns we hoped that a meal would help break the ice and help them to relax. We believed that using an action learning circle would help them with the process of topic clarification. Several of the contributors had finished a programme of study over the previous five years where they had been supported through action learning circles to use reflective practice. At the meeting things did not quite work in this way, as two other contributors also came and were concerned to check their understanding of the book. This gave us an opportunity to clarify our understanding but we did not achieve our objective and this may have deterred people who subsequently had difficulty in framing and contributing their critical incident. Despite this ten people did make their contribution and having been given the brief to discuss any aspect of their supervisory role and to use a framework of their choice for analysing the incident, they have produced work that is inspiring and optimistic.

References

Ericsson, K.A., Krampe, R. Th. & Tesch-Romer, C. (1993) The role of deliberate practice in the acquisition of expert performance. *Psychological Review* **100** (3), 363–406.

Taylor, M. (1987) Self-directed learning: more than meets the observer's eye. In *Appreciating Adults Learning: From the Learner's Perspective* (D. Boud & V. Griffin, eds), pp. 179–96. Kogan Page, London.

3.1   SUPERVISING THE DEVELOPMENT OF TECHNICAL SKILLS IN NEW STAFF

Barbara Lovelady

This incident raises the issue of adequate clinical supervision for junior members of staff when they learn technical skills in a new environment. Tripp's theoretical framework (Tripp 1993) will be used to guide my reflections and analysis of the incident. Tripp suggested that analysis can be framed in terms of practical judgement where the procedural information as to how something was done is given before describing the incident and diagnosing what happened and why as well as how it felt. He then suggests that some reflective judgement and analysis occur before moving on to evaluate how to take issues forward from that point through critical judgement and emancipation.

In this incident there was insufficient clinical supervision of the staff nurse involved and little support to facilitate her learning. Atherton (1986) described clinical supervision as the process of talking to someone else involved in the same system about what one is doing in order to do it better. Butterworth (1992) believed that models of clinical supervision can be developed in nursing which will protect and improve upon clinical practice and give nursing the necessary support it needs to mature into greater independence. He goes on to elaborate on the range of strategies in nursing for clinical supervision, which include preceptorship, mentorship, supervision of practice, peer review and support and the maintenance of standards. It is the strategy of supervision in practice which will be explored in more detail later.

This critical incident involved myself and a junior member of staff, Susan (her real name has been changed to preserve anonymity), who was newly appointed to the Cardiothoracic Intensive Care Unit (CICU). She had worked on a general medical ward for nine months since qualifying and had no previous critical care experience. Susan was on a three-week orientation course designed to introduce the principles of cardiothoracic nursing. It was a mainly theoretical course with the majority of practical input being given by mentors and more experienced staff during clinical hours on the unit. This particular incident related to one of the sessions which I had taught. The aim of the session was to teach the students how to safely set up a ventilator to receive a patient from the operating theatre. In the morning the students had been taught about theoretical aspects of ventilation by a colleague and in this afternoon session I had related that theory to practice, illustrating what we do in CICU. The students were shown how to set up the ventilator, checking their understanding of all the terms used, and then encouraged to manipulate all the dials themselves. At the end of the session, one of the ways I tested their knowledge was by setting up the ventilator incorrectly to see what they would identify as wrong and then asking them to explain its significance and remedy it. Susan noticed that the minute volume alarm settings were not set and adjusted them correctly. The whole session went well and was very positively evaluated.

Two weeks later I happened to come on to the Unit to pick up some work on a day off and was talking to Susan who proudly said she had set up her own ventilator that day albeit with a bit of a struggle to remember everything. She showed me the ventilator and as soon as I saw it I noticed that she had not set the minute volume alarms – the very problem she had previously identified and corrected in the session. Although in itself this is not a life-threatening omission, it is poor practice. If the alarms are set correctly and a problem does occur, it will often lead to earlier detection and prevention of complications.

The incident was an issue for me for many reasons. My first and overwhelming feeling was that I had failed to firmly establish in Susan's mind the basic safety principles involved in setting up a ventilator. The implication was that I had not taught the subject well during the course or that I had failed to recognise that Susan had not grasped this particular point. The second dilemma for me was how to feed back to Susan constructively, without dampening her enthusiasm or destroying her confidence. The third dilemma was the concern that nobody had noticed her omission, which raised in my mind the question of the degree of supervision present on the unit that day.

Reflecting on my own teaching, I identified that I had taken the approach of using a schema to teach (Benner 1982) consistent with the way that novices might view a new skill. This was because it is the sort of procedure where a set of rules can be applied to a given situation to provide directions for safe manipulation of the equipment. I had involved the students and encouraged them to manipulate this unfamiliar equipment appropriately in order to gain confidence. As the session had been well evaluated at the time and Susan had identified that very problem, I felt that I had achieved the session objectives and she appeared to display a good understanding at the time. However, perhaps Susan had adopted a surface approach to learning identified by Marton & Saljo (1976). This is where learning is described as memorising as opposed to the deep approach where learning is described in terms of cognition and comprehension. Fransson (1977) suggests that by making the learning situation personally relevant to the student, a deep approach is facilitated. However, giving students the scenario that a ventilator has been set up for them (incorrectly) did not seem to help with Susan's longer term learning even though in the short term this was successful. The students needed to be able to situate their learning in a relevant clinical scenario. This concept of situated cognition is validated by Brown and his co-workers (1989) who suggest that decontextualised knowledge hinders the learning process since all knowledge is situated, being in part a product of the activity, context and culture in which it is developed and used. Their evidence in addition to my own experiences in teaching have strengthened my belief that context is vital for understanding.

Decontextualised learning falls into one of the two types classified by Rogers (1969). He believes that it involves the mind only and does not involve feelings or personal meanings and is therefore quickly forgotten as it has no relevance for the whole person (Rogers 1969). Perhaps if Susan had been able to relate it to her experiences with patients on ventilators it would have been better contextualised and have had more relevance. This new knowledge and skill learned at the end of a training activity was not transferred to the normal work environment, a phenomenon previously described by Marsick & Watkins (1990). I found that people learn in the workplace through interactions with others in their daily work environment when the need to learn is greatest. This is consistent with Rogers' view that learning is most successful when motivation is high (Rogers 1969). In this critical incident, further supervised practice was required to cement Susan's knowledge and incorporate it into her own professional practice at a time when she could directly see its relevance. During preceptorship this can occur via informal learning, although in this case setting the minute volume alarms on the ventilator was reinforced by incidental learning as described by Marsick & Watkins (1990).

On reflection I believe that I had unrealistic expectations of what the students could be expected to retain. Apart from the fact that they had been bombarded with information during those first two weeks of their introductory course, most of them were still very much at the novice stage, as described by Benner using the Dreyfus and Dreyfus model of skill acquisition (Benner 1984). I think I had expected them to go from novices to competent practitioners in one step. Only after suitable coaching in the workplace is it realistic to expect the student to develop through to advanced beginner and onwards in time. It is a laudable quality in a teacher or mentor to be able to recognise the individual and unique perception of each person to understand what might be in the student's head and to recognise that it is not necessarily the same understanding as might be in theirs. This is an important factor described by Kelly (1955) and known as his personal construct theory. Had I truly considered the level of knowledge and experience of these newly appointed staff I would have had more realistic expectations.

The second issue for me was how to give constructive criticism to Susan who had obviously tried hard to get this technical skill right whilst having no previous experience of this task. I praised her for managing the rest of the ventilator correctly but added that it was important to remember these particular alarms, thus reinforcing the information given to her in the lecture. On prompting she remembered where the alarm was located but couldn't remember how to set it. I showed her again and checked her understanding, giving positive feedback when she identified clinical situations where this might be particularly important. The constructive feedback in this incident appeared to go well, with Susan stating that she would not forget that again and that she was keen to set up another one soon. This signifies growth and learning for Susan with respect to new knowledge and skills as she was gently challenged but given good support to reflect and develop. Daloz (1986) suggested that high challenge and support are the ideal combination for student growth and development. According to his theory, when challenge is low and support is variable initially (as in this case), then stasis or confirmation occurs and the student does not move on. If I had handled the feedback badly and challenged Susan without offering support, then retreat would have been inevitable and her confidence would have been destroyed consistent with Daloz's theory. As it was, the strategy of challenge sandwiched between high support was a successful one.

The final issue this incident raised for me was the lack of supervision and support given to Susan on that shift. Perhaps she had not felt able to ask someone else to check her work which is why she was so keen for me to see it as she felt more able to ask me. It is possible therefore that she felt unsupported back on the unit and very much a novice wanting to use and contextualise her new-found knowledge but trying not to bother her colleagues. It is possible that my concerns noted earlier about inadequate supervision and support on the unit that day were very real. One way to combat this could be to provide a checklist attached to the ventilators, not only to act as an *aide-mémoire* for new staff until they felt more confident but also to remind other staff in order to promote good practice. Having discussed with the students the merits of putting a checklist on the ventilator, the students welcomed the idea and so that will be provided in future. In this way the students can progress eventually to integrating practical and theoretical knowledge, the two forms of knowledge identified by Kuhn (1970), and to become self-monitoring.

Alternatively, students could have a more formal fixed period of direct supervision after the course where some particularly new aspects of the students' work must be checked. My only concern with that is that some people will grasp the principles quicker than others and then feel demotivated by over-assessment and excessive supervision when no longer needed. The ideal would probably be to manage this on a personal basis, identifying for each individual with their mentor how they will develop their potential and develop new skills. The teacher's role in the classroom could be to provide 'scaffolded instruction' (Wood *et al.* 1976) which is central to Vygotsky's notion of the zone of proximal development and involves structuring of the learning task, facilitation of student input, generalisation to less structured contexts and gradual withdrawal of the scaffold by the supervisor as learner autonomy and competence develop (Palincsar 1986). Mentors must therefore use strategies not only in order to allow students the opportunity to reflect on their experiences and social interactions from practice, but also to role model social skills necessary for the development of aesthetic and personal knowledge that the students can usefully translate into their nursing practice.

Some authors have already identified that the role conflicts experienced by clinical supervisors were perceived as inhibiting facilitation of student learning (Marrow & Tatum 1994). In this incident it is likely that the nurse who perhaps should have been supporting Susan and helping her to put her theoretical learning into practice was probably totally absorbed with her own patient care. She perhaps did not know what Susan had recently learnt and had probably not had time to ask her what she was happy to do and what she needed assistance with. The United Kingdom Central Council (1992) demands that nurses do not put patients at risk through their actions or omissions. The senior staff on the unit may have perceived that they needed to devote all of their attention to the critically ill patients as first priority and saw supporting junior staff as a secondary priority. The dilemma between being patient-centred and student-centred in clinical practice is very real and often requires a degree of negotiation, flexibility and compromise, and experience to meet the needs of all those involved.

It is noteworthy that at the time of this incident the Cardiothoracic Intensive Care Unit was very short-staffed, being nearly ten nurses below its establishment due to national recruitment problems. Although this is an increasing reality in the National Health Service, the pressure is to find ways of supporting junior staff, in the clinical area. Skill mix reviews advocate increasing the proportion of junior staff to senior staff, thus making adequate preceptorship a very real problem in practice. In this critical incident the learner was totally new to the critical care environment and theory gained during the orientation course needed to be reinforced in practice. Due to difficulties of rostering mentors and mentees together consistently when following a 12-hour shift pattern, the onus of supervision necessarily extends to others in the clinical area. Social learning and role modelling also play a crucial part in contextualising the theory learned. Marrow & Tatum (1994) also raise an uncomfortable truth about clinical supervision which is borne out by this critical incident. They suggested that although students and supervisors believe that supervision is an important learning strategy, it does not always happen in practice. Social learning may therefore be increasingly important.

Social learning

Social learning is defined by Quinn (1995) as learning which occurs when an individual learns something by observing another person doing it. That is, learning by modelling on someone else. However, I would argue that this definition is rather narrow as it appears from my observation to encompass all learning that occurs through interaction of a person with individuals or their cultural environment. In some cases it is observation of how a system works rather than an individual that provides the most powerful learning. I would still agree, however, that role modelling forms a significant part of social learning. Although this may be true, it must be recognised that the modelling may produce positive or negative learning and may or may not be a conscious process. Role modelling has long been recognised in nursing as one of the most powerful ways in which learning occurs in the clinical setting (Davies 1993) and this is supported by Melia's research (1987) which examines how student nurses learn to behave through occupational socialisation. It seems likely that this could be the mechanism for the development of aesthetic and personal nursing knowledge as described by Carper (1978) although this incident illustrates that social learning may have helped to reinforce correct behavioural skills and empirical knowledge such as setting up the ventilator correctly. It can be seen therefore that it is important to have good role models in clinical practice and even better to have clinical supervision which allows practitioners the space and time to discuss their work with support and challenge.

Wiseman (1994) identified role modelling as an effective teaching behaviour and proceeded to use Bandura's social learning theory

(Bandura 1977) to illustrate the four steps involved in learning. This framework has direct relevance to this critical incident. Bandura described the first subprocess in learning as attention to modelled behaviour but adds that there is a limit to the amount of modelled cues the observer can process at any one time. In the case of learning to set up a ventilator, perhaps the information was presented too quickly or at too complex a level, leading to only limited or fragmented learning. Bandura suggested that, if this was true, repeated presentations are necessary to produce complete and accurate learning. As Susan appeared to have grasped the principles involved in setting up the ventilator after the session, I feel that it is possibly the next subprocess necessary for learning which was the problem, i.e. retention of observed inputs by rehearsal operations or symbolic coding operations. This could have been remedied by allowing more time for supervised practice and having a checklist on the ventilator as a symbolic coding operation. The third subprocess for learning is production of a motor response whereby the student is able to demonstrate the thought processes involved in a specific action. Once the staff nurse is able to set up the ventilator and explain all the steps and their relevance to the clinical supervisor, she will have learned and internalised the information. Bandura described the final subprocess as the incentive and motivational process where modelling cues to which the observer will be attentive are selectively controlled. In this case, Susan was highly motivated to learn and very enthusiastic so I suspect her motivation was to successfully perform a new task and thus assist with her socialisation to the culture of a coronary care intensive care unit

Wiseman's study (1994) described 28 role model behaviours in the clinical setting. The list was very enlightening as it raised my awareness of the sort of behaviours I am portraying and how important they might be in setting an example for others. Perhaps this might be useful for others in the environment to look at too. It is possible there was little time to observe many role models to reinforce the theory gained before the staff nurse had to perform the as yet still fragmented task of setting up the ventilator. It is also possible that the nurse had observed a poor role model since learning the theory, who had also failed to set the minute volume alarms. After this incident I have been much more aware of how all practitioners perform this task and have been shocked and disappointed to observe that occasionally some very experienced nurses fail to set these alarms, thus promoting poor practice through negative role modeling. It is a very powerful method of teaching and one that as clinicians we must be vigilant to ensure promotes good practice by example. In this way we can promote desired behaviours and provide a clinical learning environment rich with opportunities to develop new skills.

Summary

I have reviewed this incident using Tripp's framework (1993) to help me analyse how I taught the original session, and to describe the incident and my associated feelings as well as my interpretation of what was happening. Through this process of reflection I have identified ways to improve the educational input and clinical support mechanisms for junior staff. This will be especially valuable for helping them develop new knowledge and skills in practice. It has highlighted the importance of social learning and role modelling in helping new staff become socialised to the unit. I have also become aware of the impact that new staff can have on the learning environment during clinical supervision and their need for continuous support rather than having rather *ad hoc* or unplanned experiences. This incident has also reinforced the importance of relevant knowledge, of good supervisory skills and of effective personal relationship skills for this key role (Fowler 1995, p. 33). If, as senior clinicians, we can value each practitioner as a learner and as an individual; if we can actively seek them out during the day to challenge or discuss practice; if we can communicate our advanced knowledge effectively and give constructive feedback: we will go a long way towards improving our clinical supervision and the care that our patients receive.

References

Atherton, J. S. (1986) *Professional Supervision in Group Care*. Tavistock Publications, London. Cited in: Oliver, J. (1995) Central support. *Nursing Times* **91** (26), 32–3.

Bandura, A. (1977) *Social Learning Theory*. Prentice-Hall, New Jersey.

Benner, P. (1982) From novice to expert. *American Journal of Nursing* **82** (3), 402–7.

Benner, P. (1984) *From Novice to Expert: Excellence and Power in Clinical Nursing Practice*. Addison Wesley, Menlo Park, CA.

Brown, J. S., Collins, A. Duguid, P. (1989) Situated cognition and the culture of learning. *Educational Researcher* **18** (1), 32–42.

Butterworth, T. (1992) Clinical supervision as an emerging idea in nursing. In *Clinical Supervision and Mentorship in Nursing* (T. Butterworth & J. Faugier, eds). Chapman & Hall, London.

Carper, B.A. (1978) Fundamental patterns of knowing in nursing. *Advances in Nursing Science* **1** (1), 13–23.

Daloz, L.A. (1986) *Effective Teaching and Mentoring: Realising the Transformational Power of Adult Learning Experiences*. Jossey Bass, London.

Davies, E. (1993) Clinical role modelling: uncovering hidden knowledge. *Journal of Advanced Nursing* **18** 627–36.

Ericsson, K. A., Krampe, R. Th. & Tesch-Romer, C. (1993) The role of deliberate practice in the acquisition of expert performance. *Psychological Review* **100** (3), 363–406.

Fowler, J. (1995) Nurses's perceptions of the elements of good supervision. *Nursing Times* **91** (22), 33–7.

Fransson, A. (1977) On qualitative differences in learning: IV – Effects of intrinsic motivation and extrinsic test anxiety on process and outcome. *British Journal of Educational Psychology* 47, 244–57.

Kelly, G. (1955) *The Psychology of Personal Constructs: 1 and 2*. Norton, New York.

Kuhn, T. S. (1970) *The Structure of Scientific Revolutions*. University of Chicago Press, Chicago.

Marrow, C. E. & Tatum, S. (1994) Student supervision: myth or reality? *Journal of Advanced Nursing* **19**, 1247–55.

Marsick, V. & Watkins, K. (1990) *Informal and Incidental Learning in the Workplace*. Routledge, London.

Marton, F. & Saljo, R. (1976) On qualitative differences in learning: I – Outcome and process. *British Journal of Educational Psychology* **46**, 4–11.

Melia, K. (1987) *Learning and Working: The Occupational Socialization of Nurses*. Tavistock Publications, London.

Palincsar, A. S. (1986) The role of dialogue in providing scaffolded instruction. *Educational Psychologist* **21** (1&2), 73-98.

Quinn, F.M. (1995) *The Principles and Practice of Nurse Education*, 3rd edn. Chapman & Hall, London.

Rogers, C. (1969) *Freedom to Learn*. Charles E. Merrill Publishing Company, Columbus, Ohio.

Tripp, D. (1993) *Critical Incidents in Teaching: Developing Professional Judgement*. Routledge, London.

United Kingdom Central Council for Nursing, Midwifery and Health Visiting (1992) *Code of Professional Conduct*, 3rd edn. UKCC, London.

Wiseman, R. F. (1994) Role model behaviours in the clinical setting. *Journal of Nursing Education* **33** (9), 405–10.

Wood, D. J., Bruner, J. S. & Ross, G. (1976) The role of tutoring in problem solving. *Journal of Child Psychology and Psychiatry* **17** (2), 89–100.

3.2   USING THE INTERNAL SUPERVISOR

Dave Roberts

We generally view supervision as taking place within the presence of the supervisor. In practice, though, new situations are constantly presenting us with new challenges. We have to respond to unfamiliar situations at the time by 'thinking on our feet'. Although these may be discussed with our supervisor during routine meetings, inevitably we will have to deal with the unexpected on our own. If supervision does not prepare us for times like this, then it is not working. Supervision is conceptualised here as a process of reflection between clinician, supervisor, and a specific clinical situation. As the relationship develops, the principles learned become transferable to a range of actual and potential clinical situations, where the supervisor is not present.

Using an example from my own clinical practice, I will explore some concepts from psychotherapy and the literature on reflective practice as these illuminate the way we find supervision both within ourselves and within the therapeutic relationship. I work as a mental health nurse based in a general hospital, working with patients whose primary presentation is a physical health problem. This speciality is known as liaison mental health nursing, and combines elements of direct clinical work (e.g. mental health assessment or psychotherapy) with indirect educational, supervisory and consultation elements (Roberts 1998). The clinical example is from my direct clinical work, where I was working psychotherapeutically with a patient.

The process of supervision in psychotherapy

The model developed by Patrick Casement to describe the process of supervision in psychotherapy has some interesting parallels with reflective practice (Casement 1985). He suggests that in the early stages of training there is a temptation among therapists to cling on to professional roles or theoretical bases when confronted with the strain of not knowing, i.e. the uncertainty of real clinical situations. We may compare this with the *swampy lowlands* that confront professionals in Schön's view of professional practice (Schön 1987). Casement suggests that, rather than reverting to type, the therapist should learn to take cues from the clinical material presented by the patient. Therapy then starts to become an interactive process, with the patient also responding to cues from the therapist. The first component of this interactive process is unfocused listening, which involves the therapist listening to the patient in an open and non-judgemental way. This is only possible if the therapist's anxieties are 'held' by the supervisor, in the same way that the patient's anxieties should be held by the therapist. This provides the foundation for development as an independent practitioner. As the therapist becomes more confident, the supervisor's holding function becomes internalised within the trainee therapist. There develops a capacity for spontaneous reflection within the session, alongside the internalised supervisor (Casement 1985, p.32). Therapeutic space develops between the patient and therapist, with a parallel development of reflective space within the therapist. This allows him to monitor his own practice as it takes place, in the absence of the supervisor.

In an experienced therapist practitioner, the supervisor ceases to be an internalised other, but becomes a part of the therapist, an internal supervisor, with whom s/he can have an ongoing creative dialogue. The process of therapy includes interaction with the patient. Casement suggests we extend empathy to become a form of trial identification, whereby we imagine ourselves in the place of the patient. We may then test our hypothesis by experimentation (for example, I may reflect, if the patient is feeling as I think s/he is, s/he is likely to react to my next statement this way...). This is clearly a skilled and complex activity, which requires developing self-knowledge. With practice, it becomes possible to use these two viewpoints simultaneously, the patient's and one's own, rather like following the different voices in polyphonic music. (Casement 1985, p.35). My own experience of supervision has been rich and varied. Over many years of practice, I have had supervision from psychiatrists, nurses, psychologists, counsellors and psychotherapists. I have learned a great deal about different therapeutic approaches, a variety of craft skills, and a lot about myself. Rather than having internalised one supervisor, I have integrated parts of all of them into my practice. This gives me confidence in a range of skills.

Alice's experience

The example I have chosen involves a woman in her thirties, married with a family, who developed breast cancer. This raised a number of personal issues, some immediate and practical, including how to discuss this with her children, but also deeper existential issues. To use Alice's own words:

'When I found out I had a life-threatening illness, I was shocked. But also, I felt that the time had come to decide what I thought about Life, the Universe and Everything. Otherwise I might die without knowing what I believed about things, and so die without ever having been a real person. I felt quite driven. I did a lot of reading and thinking. I did not really sleep well at this time. I would sleep for about three hours or so, and then lie in bed thinking. Gradually, as the weeks went by, I began to work out what was important in my life.'

The therapy involved working on practical issues for this patient. However, it also became a guided exploration of Alice's sense of personal meaning, both of the illness itself, and of life in general. Alice frequently had rich and colourful dreams, which seemed to provide answers to questions which were themselves only part formed. I began to see my role mainly as providing the therapeutic space and the *holding* that Casement describes occurring within therapeutic relationships. To illustrate the critical episode, I have drawn on my own thoughts, recorded soon after the session, and Alice's reflections, written independently some time later. Neither account is therefore a precise reconstruction of the events, but reflects the meaning inherent in the situation for both therapist and patient. At this meeting, Alice presented herself in a state of both excitement and perplexity, describing an experience she had had several days before:

'I went to bed as usual and fell asleep, thinking about the sort of ideas that had been preoccupying me. At about 3 am, I became suddenly awake, and found that all the thoughts I had were concentrated together into one image, which was quite overwhelming. I lay in bed, and felt the ideas with such intensity that I can only describe it by saying that the ideas seemed to burn through my veins as if my blood had turned to fire. The ideas that I had laboured over in my mind leapt to become a picture which I could see. Rather than being theoretical notions that I had acquired step by step, all of a sudden the ideas became alive, and I knew them with my body.

The image or vision that I saw consisted of two parts; one part was that I was able to perceive the forces that drive the universe. How strong they are. How constantly [they are] working without ceasing. How they are everywhere in all our lives, in all our moments of time, constantly acting and creating. The other half of the vision was that within the constant turning of the world are the ceaseless activities and doings of all the vast numbers of souls. Everyone living out their essential nature, and moving towards becoming the people they were meant to be. When a soul becomes whole, and truly and deeply itself, it becomes free, and reaches a state of ecstasy, or joy. The best part of the vision was looking at the great multitude of souls singing for joy of being truly themselves.

The most perfect form of prayer to the Creator – joy in being created. I viewed that image for a sort of timeless moment, and eventually passed into sleep.'

At the time both Alice and I were perplexed by this. I felt some excitement at this new development, but neither of us yet understood what it meant for her or the therapy. The internalised psychiatric supervisor in me wondered if it was a sign of incipient mental illness. It would have been easy to be overcautious. I could have deferred any decisions until I had discussed the situation with my supervisor. However, I realised that my immediate reaction was too important to appear vague or confused. My own experience of supervision suggested that much of its value was in the supervisor accepting what was presented in an open and non-judgemental way. My supervisors had not responded by saying either 'I know what this means' or 'I don't know what this means'. Rather they had asked, 'What do you think this means?' Experience is rooted in the personal meaning we ascribe to it. If experience ceases to have meaning, or if the meaning is substantially incongruent with the experience of others, then mental illness is a possibility. Alice's experience had congruence with her previous, rich dream world and it seemed laden with symbolic meaning. It was hard to identify with, as I had never had a waking vision, and it seemed more like a dream than anything else. Until it became clearer what the meaning was for Alice, I felt I must suspend my own reaction, for fear of prejudicing her understanding of what it meant to her. I needed to clarify how she felt about the experience. Alice herself had some anxieties, as she asked me:

'People don't normally experience this sort of thing, do they?'

In my experience, when people ask what's normal, they are usually worried they are abnormal. Often this takes the form of fears of losing control or going mad in the face of a new, unfamiliar experience. It felt most important that she should not feel that I was afraid or anxious, which would undermine her sense of control. By my remaining calm and accepting, and focusing on her interpretation of the experience and its meaning, the therapy would hold her and enhance her own ability to contain her feelings. My response was to say that comparisons with other people's experience would probably not help, as this was clearly an unusual event. It was, however, very real for Alice, and could have a lot of personal meaning. But new experiences can be disconcerting, so I asked her if she was frightened, if she felt in control.

'The next day, I found the experience had been so powerful that I was tired out. Also, my interior world was becoming so strong, that it seemed as if it might be overcoming the external world, and this was frightening, as it seemed only a few steps away from mental chaos. So I let the vision go – it wasn't possible to live at that level of intensity for very long.'

So the intensity of the experience rather than the experience itself was frightening and Alice decided to let go of the feelings it engendered, thereby remaining in control. This meant Alice could further reflect on the experience from a position of some detachment, without feeling overwhelmed. The spectre of mental illness faded into the background, I suspect for both of us. Unexpectedly at this stage I was helped by the patient to reflect on the meaning of this session for me as a therapist. It is only possible to respond to opportunities like this if the therapist engages in unfocused listening and does not respond automatically or in a formulaic way. Alice realised her experience was unusual. She asked me how I could continue to work with people if they made little progress, or just accepted life without question. This made me reflect on my own experiences both as a therapist and as a person. Although I had never had an experience like Alice's, I once had a dream that showed me a vision of a large, single-roomed building. It was intricately carved inside and out, with thin walls but tremendously strong. I came to realise this was a vision of myself, complete as I could be, a vision of my whole self. By sharing this with Alice I saw that 'personal visions' of our potential, in whatever form they take, indicate how we can all change for the better and become whole. It is the very ability to have a vision of human potential that enables therapists to continue in their work. It was possible for us both to talk about this, not because we shared the same experience, but because we could interpret the other's experience in a way that was meaningful for us. This was based on our trust in the therapeutic relationship, which we had both worked to create. What is possible to disclose in therapy may not necessarily be shared outside of it. Alice's next comment made me realise that the *holding* or *containing* function of therapy made it safe to discuss sensitive experiences:

'I'm not going to tell everyone about this. They probably would not understand.'

Reflections

This session was really challenging but, like many other sessions with this patient, was stimulating and positive. It would have been too easy to panic or take an over-cautious view of her experience which would have denied the potential in the situation for her and for the therapy. Psychoanalysis, a branch of psychotherapy with its base in medicine, is an example of a profession which claims to be grounded in technical rationality but which in practice is more of an art, where skill or artistry is learned through a reflective process (Schön 1983). The system of learning in psychoanalysis involves a complex system of reflections between supervisor and trainee, trainee and patient that Schön has described as a hall of mirrors (Schön 1987). This session involved a reflective process involving the therapist, the patient, and the internal supervisor. Schön suggests that it is necessary for people working in conceptually complex fields like psychiatry and psychotherapy to communicate within the same frame in order for their discussions to have any real meaning. Understanding can only take place across frames when a capacity for frame reflection has developed (Schön 1987).

In order to really understand someone, we have to suspend pre-conceptions and resist categorising them and their experience. We can achieve this by *unfocused listening* which allows us to hear what they are really saying (Casement 1985). We must then develop an ability to understand their experience by referring to our own; by developing a capacity to reflect across frames of reference. Jones (1998) describes how, viewed from Heidegger's phenomenological perspective, caregiving is a meeting of two worlds of experience. The resulting connection is termed *co-constituency*, that is, experience jointly constituted. We can only do this if we have confidence in our ability to contain the uncertainty and anxiety that arise when we expose ourselves to the experiences of others. Reflecting now some time after the event, I can best understand Alice's experience as a spiritual one. Spirituality is poorly handled in our materialistic, rationalistic society. It is not surprising therefore that Alice decided not to share it with many people. This experience could only have meaning in Alice's own terms. So, on reflection, what did this experience mean?

> 'Later I tried to judge the experience. Was it valuable or was it a sign of mental instability and not to be trusted? I judged it by its effects. It gave me a feeling of great confidence, energy, and security, and made me feel more connected and involved with people, and more responsible and sensitive towards them as individuals. Almost as if, having sharpened senses, I was seeing people as they really were for the first time.'

What were the sources of supervision in this meeting? I was not aware of any one internalised supervisor. Rather, processes of supervision over a period of time had combined to give me both confidence in myself, and confidence in the capacity of therapeutic relationships to be containing and therapeutic. The role of the relationship itself was pivotal. Alice provided a form of supervision by giving her own meaning to the experience. She then acted as supervisor for me by helping me to reflect on the meaning of such experiences for the process of therapy. In turn, my responses enabled the patient to internalise her own sense of personal containment, giving her the space to reflect and find her own meaning. Kemmis (1985) has observed that by defining experience through the reflective learning process we are potentially redefining human experience and societal norms. By keeping our minds open when sharing the wonderfully rich diversity of human experience, we not only help our patients and ourselves to gain a deeper understanding of life, but we also help to define human experience itself.

'As regards the meeting, I think, in retrospect, I am very grateful that you were able to accept what I told you on its own merits, and that it was not reduced to fit into some theory of behaviour. This probably required quite a leap of the imagination! I felt your sensitivity was an expression of respect towards me, which allowed me the confidence to accept the experience in a very positive way. The memory of the image has remained a sort of anchor in my thoughts, and a moment of personal revelation.'

References

Casement, P. (1985) *On Learning from the patient*. Routledge, London.

Jones, A. (1998) Remembering Mair Jones (the co-constituency of care giving). *International Journal of Palliative Nursing*, 4 (1), 44–7.

Kemmis, S. (1985) Action research and the politics of reflection. In *Reflection: Turning Experience into Learning* (D. Boud, R. Keogh & D. Walker, eds), pp. 139–63. Kogan Page, London.

Roberts, D. (1998) Making the connections to aid mental health. *Nursing Times*, 94 (15), 50–2.

Schön, D. (1983) *The Reflective Practitioner: How Professionals Think in Action*. Basic Books, New York.

Schön, D. (1987) *Educating the Reflective Practitioner*. Jossey Bass, Oxford.

3.3   LESSONS OF EXPERIENCE: WORKING WITH STUDENTS IN COMMUNITY MIDWIFERY PRACTICE

Lorna Cowan

'Education is something we neither give nor do to our students. Rather, it is a way we stand in relation to them.' (Daloz 1986)

This paper is based on an early mentoring experience I initially regarded as a disaster. I have returned to this experience over the years to examine what went wrong and it has helped me to appreciate the complexity of the mentoring relationship. Drawing on the work of Daloz (1986) I identify three key areas which appear crucial in the mentoring relationship and indeed the therapeutic relationship in (midwifery) practice:

- Establish a relationship
- Provide a framework
- Address your concerns

These three areas are explored in relation to my example of inexperienced mentoring and suggestions are made for good practice.

The critical incident

This critical incident briefly describes one of my earliest experiences working as a mentor after four years of varied midwifery practice. I was working as a team midwife and was asked to work as a mentor for an undergraduate midwifery student for a module. I shall call this student Amy. Our work together involved working 120 hours over a 12-week term. How this should be achieved was for us to sort out together.

Working as a team midwife was often intense and unpredictable. It included: periods of 24 hours on call, intensive spells on delivery suite caring for labouring women and their partners, providing clinics for pregnant women, and community visiting to families with a new baby. There was little opportunity for Amy to work alone, therefore we were in intense contact with each other for periods of 6–24 hours.

Initially I was delighted to have a student and enjoyed sharing my knowledge and skills with her. However, I began to feel uncomfortable when I found Amy increasingly critical of my practice and less able in her own practice than she had led me to expect. I became increasingly concerned when Amy appeared generally depressed and exhausted; she didn't always relate well with women and I found her painfully slow at practical tasks. She tended to cry when I tried to discuss her practice with her. Things became worse when Amy became very upset while we were caring for a woman in labour whose labour was becoming difficult and medicalised. Amy left the delivery suite and went home. I felt this was inappropriate and generally resented the time and energy I was forced to give Amy during busy times at work.

I discussed my concerns with a course tutor and lecturer–practitioner, and Amy and I met her personal tutor. It was generally agreed that I should be more supportive. No formal plan was made for our on-going work together. I did my utmost to be supportive but found a lot of tension between being supportive and addressing my concerns about Amy's performance in practice. Things eventually deteriorated to the point where Amy would phone in on the days she had agreed to work. She would be clearly upset, say she couldn't come in and refuse all offers of further meetings. Amy passed that module on the strength of her written work but eventually left the course.

Establishing a relationship

Establishing a relationship is time consuming. It is particularly difficult when you are already busy with clinical work. However, it is essential to providing a good learning experience for a student. The aim is to see the world through the eyes of your student and then to lead them on from there (Rogers 1983; Daloz 1986). If you can develop this empathy with your student, she will feel that she can relate to you and will be more likely to learn from you. An ability to quickly develop an empathetic relationship seems to be the mark of an effective mentor/teacher and Daloz gives examples of this in his book. From my own experience of being a student and a patient in a variety of contexts it is the single most important quality in a mentor, teacher, midwife, doctor or therapist. Similarly, student nurses rate good interpersonal skills as the most important quality in a mentor (Marriott 1991; Brown 1993). I think there are two main reasons why I did not establish this sort of relationship with Amy.

First, I did not invest enough focused time on the relationship. I thought it was enough to ask her some questions and have some social chat at opportune moments, for example in the car on the way to a community visit or while grabbing a quick lunch. I now feel it is essential that some time be deliberately allocated to making some initial assessment of the student, when you ask open questions and really listen to what is being said. What brought her into midwifery? Has she any idea what she wants to learn during your time together? The amount of time to be spent on this and the breadth and depth of your enquiry relate to the nature of the mentoring relationship. Obviously it is much more superficial if you are working with a student for a matter of days rather than weeks or months. If you invest time in this, the student immediately feels valued and you can tailor your future interactions to her needs. I didn't find any time to do this properly with Amy and this no doubt contributed to her feeling undervalued and misunderstood by me. No wonder I found her increasingly critical of my practice. I expected her to see clinical situations as I did and became frustrated when she would latch on to some seemingly trivial detail. However, as students learn, they move from seeing discrete elements to seeing the whole (Benner 1984) and from seeing things as black or white to accepting that most things are grey (Perry 1968). It is the mentor who must try to see things from the student's point of view.

The second problem I had was that I was very conscious of my own performance. I felt very conscious of the impression I was making, and of the knowledge I wanted to share with Amy. This makes it more difficult to focus on the student's needs. This appears to be a particular problem until you feel comfortable with yourself in the role of mentor. The problem is compounded in clinical practice by having a patient as the primary focus of care. In addition, in midwifery practice I may be caring for a mother, a baby and other family members in a rapidly changing or emotionally charged situation. However, as I have become more experienced as a mentor (and as a midwife), I have found it easier to focus on the student's needs as well as being able to deal with increasingly complex clinical situations. Benner (1984) describes this developing expertise in detail.

Amy's inability to always relate well to patients probably reflected her inexperience. Her mind would be totally focused on learning new tasks. The mentor needs to know what is reasonable to expect from a student at their particular stage. Written guidelines and support from an experienced mentor or teacher can help new mentors with this.

Suggestions for practice

- Set time aside to assess the student at the beginning of a mentoring relationship.
- Spend more time analysing your student's performance and less on your own.
- Recognise that you have to learn to become an effective mentor.

Providing a framework

It is useful to provide a framework for students, and the concept of a framework can be applied on a number of levels to this critical incident. It can be used to:

- Describe the general orientation of a student to a clinical area
- Explain the type of work experience on offer (e.g. antenatal clinics, intra-partum care, postnatal community visiting)
- Describe the geography of the work place (e.g. health centres, delivery suite, community)
- Provide specific guidelines for students (e.g. what to wear, where to meet, whether to bring a packed lunch)

Ideally all this information could be given in a written welcome pack for each practice area as lots of verbal information at the beginning of a placement may not be remembered. Providing a welcome pack is another example that an initial investment in time promotes effective mentoring.

In Amy's case a more fundamental framework was also required. We needed to build a framework to structure the whole work experience. In common with an increasing number of students whose courses are based on adult learning theories which stress student-centred and self-directed learning, Amy came with no pre-planned timetable. The overall number of days she worked, where she worked and when she worked (to a minimum of 120 hours) were open to negotiation. I understood student-centred and self-directed learning to mean that Amy was largely responsible for planning her own work experience. However, I now feel that it is absolutely essential that a mentor be actively involved in this process. The mentor might be a personal tutor or course leader rather than a midwife in practice like myself. A mentor must be involved because Amy did not have sufficient experience of team midwifery to plan a realistic timetable. I now feel she underestimated the stress of learning in the context of team midwifery and we verbally agreed on an over-ambitious plan. This sort of plan is often called a learning contract and as the term implies it should be clearly documented. It is common for students to be overambitious, and it must therefore be accepted that the learning contract may need to be modified throughout the work experience. The mentor should moderate a hopelessly over-ambitious plan to prevent exhaustion and demoralisation which inhibit learning (Daloz 1986; Rogers 1986).

The 24-hour on-calls were a particular problem for Amy. It is not surprising that she would feel overwhelmed trying to care for labouring women for up to 24 hours. It was sometimes overwhelming for experienced midwives and is a practice that has since been abandoned. As Amy's mentor I needed to make sure her basic needs such as sleep, food and relaxation were being met as these are prerequisite to personal growth/ learning (Maslow 1970).

The most effective mentors are able to modify the framework regularly at a sophisticated level. For example, the mentor needs to be aware of areas of practice that students feel uncomfortable with and that they may consequently try to avoid. Sometimes students are aware of their own difficult areas and will tell you that they need extra support; however, sometimes the avoidance may not even be conscious. I became aware that Amy had a particular problem coping with abnormal labour when she avoided it in a very concrete way: she walked out of the delivery suite while we were caring for a woman whose labour became abnormal. I will come back to dealing with potential conflict in the next section but want to highlight here the need for mentors to be constantly assessing the student and noting areas where development is required. Claxton (1984) recognises that the most profound learning often occurs when the student feels most uncomfortable when deeply held beliefs are challenged. The mentor may need to help the student confront difficult areas and amend the learning contract accordingly.

The concept of a framework for the mentoring relationship itself is also invaluable for the mentor and student. Some details of how the relationship will be structured can be written into the learning contract. This includes where, when and for how long key meetings such as initial assessment, mid-term review and final evaluation will take place. This helps the student plan for these and makes them a priority for the mentor. Some sort of agreement about the day-to-day running of the relationship should also be formalised. For example, agree where and when a brief daily review can occur. When working with Amy I tended to raise areas of concern while driving between community visits. This disadvantaged Amy because she was trapped in my space and had no time to prepare, and disadvantaged me because I could not focus properly on our interaction. As soon as our clinical work finished Amy would go home. It would have been much better to plan a five minute chat in the office at the end of each working day, even better if Amy had spent some time on reflection while I did paperwork. Then if either of us had concerns, an on-going plan could have been made. This highlights again that effective mentoring requires dedicated time and attention from the mentor and is not done well if it only happens informally around clinical work. Most mentoring does of course occur like this, but an underlying framework is essential for students with problems.

Suggestions for practice

- Prepare a welcome pack to introduce students to your area.
- At an initial meeting write a learning contract which includes the where and when of clinical work and key meetings.
- The mentor and student should regularly review the student's progress using an agreed format.

Address your concerns

I found it difficult to discuss my concerns with Amy without her becoming upset, sometimes to the extent that she would need to go home. This was obviously an extreme reaction but it is always difficult to maintain a supportive stance towards your student whilst also tackling worrying aspects of their work. Most of the literature on mentorship stresses the supportive aspect of the role but little advice is given on dealing with unsatisfactory performance. Similarly, Amy's personal tutor advised me to be more supportive of Amy but no advice was given on how to appropriately address my concerns.

Daloz (1986) recognises that mentors need to challenge students to help them to grow. Challenge might include: pushing their boundaries, reflecting back to them how they appear in practice, suggesting alternative ways of thinking or doing things and questioning their assumptions. He recognises that the student must also feel supported or they may perceive challenge as so threatening that they regress. This results in the student performing less competently than they are able and employing more rigid modes of thinking. Amy did seem to find my attempts to discuss her practice very threatening and I seemed unable to help her to feel supported once she felt threatened. What this experience has taught me is that it is essential to demonstrate support for students before you can challenge them. One of the most effective ways of providing support is to establish a relationship and provide a framework as I have described above. Daloz (1986) also suggests expressing positive expectations and sharing ourselves. Sharing ourselves resonates with Rogers' (1983) concept of congruence. Rogers also recognises that there are two elements in the teaching relationship. The first is what he describes as maintaining a positive regard for students which is similar to providing support, i.e. expressing positive expectations and helping to contain the student's experience. This is balanced by the teacher remaining congruent, i.e. the teacher is true to herself and is prepared to express her feelings and opinion even if it is in conflict with the student's view. Rogers (1983) suggests that the student is most likely to grow if they perceive positive regard and congruence from the teacher. If the mentor is articulate about her personal values and demonstrates them in practice, she helps the student assimilate professional values in a powerful way. This is an important aspect of education for professional practice (Jarvis 1983).

It is much easier to comfortably express your own opinion if you have good self-esteem. (Burns 1979). As I have gained experience in midwifery and mentoring and reflected upon this experience, I have become more confident and articulate about my practice. Consequently I no longer find students questioning my practice as irritating and threatening, as I did with Amy, but rather as an opportunity to share my practice.

Students' self-esteem also affects their ability to learn (Burns 1979). Positive self-esteem enables the student to cope with the stress of learning situations and respond positively to the challenge of being questioned and being presented with new ideas. Gender may also influence one's ability to respond to challenge. Belenky *et al.* (1986) found that women responded best to supportive methods of teaching and could find a challenging approach debilitating. Amy's self-esteem might already have been low at the time she was working with me or she may have found my approach incompatible with her learning style. Also, she was unlikely to have found me congruent as I was trying to appear positive while actually feeling very worried about her performance in practice. It is not surprising that this was not a mentoring relationship that would promote growth.

The way in which you challenge a student is also vital. The timing and the place are important. For example, do not broach potentially threatening subjects in the car on the way to visiting patients as I did with Amy. It is better to wait until your prearranged times outlined in the learning contract or to arrange a time to discuss a specific issue, thereby giving the student some time to prepare.

What you say is important. Focus on concrete behaviour rather than generalisations. For example, rather than saying, 'you don't appear to be coping' say, 'I think we need to look at the learning contract again as you went home earlier than I expected on Saturday. Do you have any thoughts about how we should organise your workload?' It is much easier to use specific examples if you have a written learning contract and you document your work together. This only needs to be brief notes in your diary. I had no documentation of my plan with Amy and wished I had kept more notes in my work diary. When there is conflict within a mentoring relationship, good assessment, planning, documentation and evaluation are invaluable to both the student and the mentor.

The very notion of mentors assessing students and documenting the relationship has been questioned because it can compromise the supportive aspect of mentorship (Morton-Cooper & Palmer 1993). However, I hope that I have demonstrated that some sort of assessment is integral to mentorship. Moreover, the mentor working alongside a student in clinical practice is best placed to assess a student's performance in practice. As performance in practice is an essential component of any assessment strategy for professional qualification, it seems sensible to include the mentors' assessment in any assessment strategy.

Suggestions for practice

- Value your opinion and be prepared to express it.
- Challenge students at an appropriate time and place.
- Be specific in your feedback.

I hope it has become obvious that the mentor is also a student: she is learning how to become an effective mentor. During this critical incident I needed support to bolster my crumbling self-esteem and I needed to feel that someone had really heard my concerns. I needed help to formulate a plan to deal effectively with a difficult situation. This could have been based on the existing assessment strategy. I also needed help to understand why Amy might have found me threatening. There is therefore a need for those learning to become mentors to receive effective mentorship themselves. In midwifery this could be incorporated into the supervisory process providing the supervisor has the requisite skills.

I have come to realise that effective mentorship uses the same skills that are essential to effective midwifery practice. These are the ability:

- To make a thorough assessment
- To use this assessment to formulate an appropriate plan
- To implement and continuously evaluate the plan
- To document what happens, and to involve others when necessary

To make it really special, maintain a stance that says: 'I am here to serve this woman and/or student to the best of my ability and I am not frightened to share myself in the process'.

References

Belenky, M.F., Clinchy, B.M., Goldberger, N.R. & Tarule. J. (1986) *Women's Ways of Knowing: The Development of Self, Voice and Mind.* Basic Books, New York. Quoted in: Merriam, S. & Caffarella, R. (1991) *Learning in Adulthood.* Jossey Bass, San Francisco.

Benner, P. (1984) *From Novice to Expert: Excellence and Power in Clinical Nursing Practice.* Addison-Wesley, Menlo Park, CA.

Brown, G. (1993) Accounting for power: nurse teachers' and students' perceptions of power in their relationship. *Nurse Education Today*, 13, 111–20.

Burns, R.B. (1979) *The Self-concept: Theory, Measurement, Development and Behaviour*. Longman, London.

Claxton, G. (1984) *Live and Learn*. Harper & Row, London.

Daloz, L.A. (1986) *Effective Teaching and Mentoring*. Jossey Bass, San Francisco.

Jarvis, P. (1983) *Professional Education*. Croom Helm, London.

Marriott, A. (1991) The support, supervision and instruction of nurse learners in clinical areas: a literature review. *Nurse Education Today* 11, 261–9.

Maslow, A.H. (1970) *Motivation and Personality*, 2nd edn. Harper & Row, New York.

Merriam, S. & Caffarella, R. (1991) *Learning in Adulthood*. Jossey Bass, San Francisco.

Morton-Cooper, A. & Palmer, A. (1993) *Mentorship and Preceptorship. A Guide to Support Roles in Clinical Practice*. Blackwell Science, Oxford.

Perry, W.G. (1968) *Forms of Intellectual and Ethical Development in the College Years: A Scheme*. Holt, Rinehart & Winston, New York. Cited in Daloz, L.A. (1986) *Effective Teaching and Mentoring*. Jossey Bass, San Francisco.

Rogers, A. (1986) *Teaching Adults*. Open University Press, Milton Keynes.

Rogers, C. (1983) *Freedom to Learn for the 80s*. Merrill Macmillan Publishing Co., New York.

3.4   ESTABLISHING SUPPORT WHEN SUPERVISING CLINICAL COLLEAGUES

Charlotte Chesson

Whilst working as a team leader and supervisor to Ann, a more junior staff nurse in my team, I encountered a management issue that caused me to reflect on my role and to question my attitudes with regard to supervision. I had returned to work from time away whilst Ann had just gone off duty. The incident arose on reading Ann's care plans and documentation for one of her patients. We had agreed that in my absence Ann would take responsibility for this patient. This included assessing his needs and planning his care with him, his loved ones and the other health care staff who would also be involved. Yet this paperwork appeared to be incomplete in that Ann had not carried out a comprehensive assessment of the patient's needs even though he had been an in-patient for several days whilst Ann was caring for him. A scant care plan was provided that did little to inform subsequent carers of what nursing care was planned or required for the patient. Ann had been successful in taking on this responsibility independently in the past, but her current work was of a poor standard, which was a significant deterioration from her previous achievements. This change in her work worried me, as it seemed that she had lost motivation and enthusiasm for her clinical practice and possibly even for her commitment to patients. I was disappointed because Ann had initially been very motivated and had put a lot of effort into her work since our last supervisory session. Previously I had believed that she had responded well to that session and was happy at work. Now I felt let down. I was conscious that I was annoyed but also that I felt guilty for having these thoughts and feelings about Ann. I decided that I should meet with her to discuss my concerns but was anxious that I had prejudged her apparent 'loss of form'.

Discussion and analysis

To explore this incident I used the work of the American psychotherapist and educator Carl Rogers (1961) whose work can be extended to helping relationships in other professions which share a common intention. Rogers offers a theoretical framework for viewing interpersonal relationships and identifies some specific characteristics whereby learning can be facilitated. He suggests that 'realness' or 'genuineness' is an essential attribute that facilitators require in order to be effective. Rogers describes the facilitator as being real when s/he enters into a relationship without presenting a front to others and is in touch with their feelings and capable of communicating these to others if appropriate. However, using Rogers' (1983) argument, by acknowledging and owning the feelings as mine rather than caused by Ann, there is no need to impose them on her. In this way I can separate my annoyance about Ann's work from my feelings towards her as a person. Thus, I could feel angry about the poor quality of her work whilst maintaining a genuine concern and interest in her as a colleague. Rogers recognises the natural tendency to judge the person by their work and thus apportion blame, locking both parties into a negative relationship. If I had allowed my negative judgements and assumptions about Ann to have surfaced, either verbally or non-verbally, she could have become angry or upset at being treated unfairly and have retreated from any discussion. Even by verbalising my feelings by saying something like 'I find these care plans frustrating. I am methodical and find it difficult to follow them', I can be presenting a façade if I feel judgemental. The process of acting in a truly genuine manner is extremely difficult even when trying wholeheartedly to do so (Rogers 1983, p.127). Later, Rogers argues that *realness* or congruence is more effective than presenting a façade, which covers the negative feelings and implies an interest. Congruence between feelings and acts, he argues, is central to any relationship, which can be deepened by such risk taking (Rogers & Stevens 1991). In the relationship with Ann, I should try to be honest and share my feelings of distress that I am disappointed and find it uncomfortable to say this to her. Consequently, I feel remote from her and have difficulty understanding her feelings and motivation that I do not wish to happen. Saying this causes me to feel both expectant and apprehensive but it is also showing that I am genuinely seeking to understand her and to be in touch with her.

By trying to be genuine and to create a successful, helping relationship that promotes personal growth and development, the facilitator is able to prize, accept and trust the student or client. As a result s/he is communicating a caring attitude towards the person in a non-possessive way and demonstrates an acceptance of the other as a trustworthy and separate individual with all the normal human frailties. By accepting Ann's feelings (perhaps her apathy) I am communicating that I am accepting her weaknesses as much as her efforts. Often it is difficult to acknowledge that we are holding such ambivalent feelings towards each other, but it is only by accepting them that we can build healthy and productive relationships that allow people to grow. The process of *unconditional positive regard* requires unreserved trust and acceptance, which precludes judgement or censorship (Rogers & Stevens 1991, p.94). Achieving this state of mind in professional and managerial relationships, particularly when working in busy and often stressful clinical settings, is difficult, and Rogers & Stevens (1991) acknowledge this, arguing that it can only be achieved by developing a profound trust in the human organism. This includes having a faith in oneself and being able to deal with one's own human frailties. Whilst this is a personally challenging and lifelong goal to work towards, it also offers opportunities and rewards for both participants in the relationship and hopefully for the rest of the team, as well as our patients.

Epilogue

This critical incident was written some years ago and as such 'frames' a point in my development as a practitioner and particularly as a manager. It is an example of what Schön (1991) describes as reflection-on-action as opposed to reflection-in-action. Reflection-on-action occurs after an incident and focuses on the development of the practitioner's skills via a consideration and analysis of the event and the knowledge that the practitioner used. Reflection-in-action occurs during clinical practice and can therefore have an immediate effect on the clinician's thoughts and decision-making processes and their subsequent actions.

The impetus for this reflection was a negative feeling. Boyd & Fales (1983) state that this is often the case and describe this as an 'inner discomfort'. Boud *et al.* (1994) suggest that a loss of confidence or disillusionment may act as a trigger for the reflective process. At the time that I initially explored this incident I was an inexperienced team leader and I lacked confidence and experience in managing other members of staff and their performance. This was in direct contrast to my clinical skills in managing patient care, an area in which I had faith in my own judgement and ability to manage relationships. Thus my under-confidence acted as a prompt for the reflective process which was then focused on trying to make sense of the situation and how I should approach Ann in order for us to work well together and resolve problems. Benner (1984) suggests that events that appear to be mundane are worthy of re-examination and can constitute critical incidents in their own right. On the surface of things the incident appears to be mundane and inconsequential, yet conversely my development in this area was central to my development as a manager. I needed to consider how I worked with others and what were my values and beliefs in this area. I wanted to work with Ann to facilitate her development and learning so that she could think critically about her own performance and make positive changes and improvements. Brookfield (1986) describes the role of the facilitator to adult learners as involving prompting learners to analyse their behaviours and assumptions, to consider new ideas, values and alternatives and to perceive themselves as proactive beings. He describes discussion as a useful teaching method, and posing questions may be a part of this discourse. Brookfield (1986) states that as facilitators we cannot force people to think critically but we can try to prompt, nurture and encourage this process. He suggests that critical questioning can assist in this process, i.e. questioning designed to elicit the assumptions underlying our thoughts and actions and to prompt reflection and analysis rather than just to obtain information (Brookfield 1987). This can assist in reflecting back learners' attitudes, rationalisations, and habitual ways of acting and thinking so they can view their motivations, actions and justifications as others may (Brookfield 1986). Brookfield's ideas relate closely to the work of Daloz (1986) who describes successful mentors as acting as a *mirror* to their students. Brookfield (1986) describes the activities involved in challenging adults to consider alternative points of view and beliefs as uncomfortable and painful at times.

I wanted to act as a facilitator in my interaction with Ann and I needed to consider my feelings towards her if I was to adopt this role. This approach is most akin to clinical supervision and would therefore only be successful in exploring the causes of her poor performance, and her insight into this, if these issues were on her agenda. However, her apparent failing gave rise to concerns for me as a manager as they could result in a poor experience for the patient. I realised that if my initial interchange with her proved to be unproductive I would need to take a more top-down approach to managing this issue in the form of management supervision. Getting a sensitive balance between these approaches was the cause of my *inner discomfort*.

Morton-Cooper & Palmer (1993) note that supervision has become too specifically focused on mainly punitive and monitoring elements in the field of general nursing. The challenge is to use professional judgement to manage the situation and intervention appropriately and give constructive feedback to staff in order to address poor performance in a sensitive and humanistic manner.

I believe that the process of reflection and writing the critical incident gave me insight into the 'theories-in-use' that guided my thoughts. Argyris and Schön (1978) classify action theories into theories-in-use and espoused theories. Espoused theories, they suggest, are action theories to which practitioners claim allegiance whilst theories-in-use are those which govern and affect practice and are observable. Argyris & Schön describe how these theories may be discrepant, but practitioners may lack insight into this anomaly in their behaviour. I believe that I was thoughtful and striving to be fair to Ann via my deliberations and that I was using reflection to critically examine my practice and as such acting as my own internal challenge and support.

References

Argyris, C. & Schön, D.A. (1978) *Organisational Learning*. Addison-Wesley, Massachusetts.

Benner, P. (1984) *From Novice to Expert: Excellence and Power in Clinical Nursing Practice*. Addison-Wesley, Menlo Park, CA.

Boud, D., Keogh, R. & Walker, D. (1994) *Reflection: Turning Experience into Learning*. Kogan Page, London.

Boyd, E.M. & Fales, A.W. (1983) Reflective learning: key to learning from experience. *Journal of Humanistic Psychology* 23 (2), 99-117.

Brookfield, S.D. (1986) *Understanding and Facilitating Adult Learning*. Open University Press, Milton Keynes.

Brookfield, S.D. (1987) *Developing Critical Thinkers*. Open University Press, Milton Keynes.

Daloz, L. (1986) *Effective Teaching and Mentoring: Realizing the Transformational Power of Adult Learning Experiences*. Jossey Bass, San Francisco.

Morton-Cooper, A. & Palmer, A. (1993) *Mentoring and Preceptorship*. Blackwell Science, Oxford.

Rogers, C. (1961) *On Becoming a Person: A Therapist's View of Psychotherapy*. Constable and Co., London.

Rogers, C. (1983) *Freedom to Learn for the 80s*. Charles E. Merrill Publishing Company, Ohio.

Rogers, C. & Stevens, B. (1991) *Person to Person, the Problem of Being Human*. Condor Books, Souvenir Press, London.

Schön, D.A. (1991) *The Reflective Practitioner*, 2nd edn, Jossey Bass, San Francisco.

3.5 THE 'MESSY MIRROR': CONFRONTING PERSONAL ISSUES IN FIELDWORK PLACEMENTS

Mary Kavanagh

One of the hardest, and yet potentially most rewarding, experiences as a fieldwork educator has been to help students on placement. This has been not only to develop their skills as future occupational therapists, but also to face up to and address their own personal fears and insecurities in dealing with clients' life issues – particularly those that mirror the students' own. It has been my experience that, when working in a mental health setting, often with younger clients issues crop up which can bear an uncanny and sometimes unsettling resemblance to the students' own personal struggles. These issues may include alcohol abuse, sexual abuse and eating disorders and maybe more complex examples. Others deal with loss of relationships, facing exams, and depression. Occupational therapists work from a frame of reference which is basically client-centred, being with the client or patient where they are mentally and physically, and looking at working with them in a way that is empowering to the latter. It is often the boundaries around this that students find the most complex and hardest to deal with on a personal level. I want to explore the issues around this 'messy mirror' as one student described it. I feel that the personal development of self, the *therapeutic use of self* as defined by Schwartzberg (1993), is where the student learns to develop further their qualities of understanding, caring and empathy. This is a vital part of placement experience. Yet this personal development is often unacknowledged by the grading system within university marking guidelines for placements. Furthermore, it is viewed by some as a potential disadvantage to achieving competence, for fear that acknowledging those areas may be seen as weakness and failure. There are no straightforward answers to this.

What can aid the process are a number of factors. These are:

- Students' openness to, and honesty about, experiencing distress and uncomfortable feelings
- Their ability to look beyond distress to a likely explanation
- Their willingness to problem-solve for ways to deal with the distress
- Their ability to work in a professional way

I want to use an episode from practice to illustrate the potential crises and opportunities that can arise from a painful encounter. This took place with a client whose life experience mirrored that of a trainee therapist. In the process I have used a model of reflection to look at the way the situation was pondered upon, and resolved (Fish *et al.* 1991).

Four strands of reflection (Fish *et al.* 1991)
- The factual – Setting the scene, telling the story, pinpointing critical incidents
- The retrospective – Looking back at the events, seeking meanings and patterns, reviewing process, outcome and personal strands
- The substratum – Examination of the hidden agenda: assumptions, beliefs, attitudes and values underpinning the event
- The connective – Implications: for practice, for personal learning; are conceptions or assumptions challenged?

The factual strand: The mirror encountered

Elizabeth was a mature student who came to the mental health unit on an 11-week placement in the first term of the last year of her three-year course. She had had two previous placements, one on an orthopaedic ward, and one in a learning disabilities unit. Normally Elizabeth would have spent all her time working with one therapist, shadowing her work initially and then taking on a caseload of her own for at least the last half of the placement. During her placement this is what did happen. In week 5 of her placement during a review, I suggested that she saw a patient called Ann, who had been admitted with severe depression following a series of losses in her life. These losses had included the death of her mother, the closure of the firm where she worked and the loss of a good friend who had left the area. Elizabeth initially agreed to see Ann to assess her needs and to look at engaging her in the group programme on the ward. In the supervision session, the interview with Ann was discussed. Elizabeth mentioned that Ann had been very tearful and distressed and did not want to talk about anything other than how upset she was over her mother's death. Elizabeth had therefore not stayed with her very long, and had not discussed the programme with her.

The retrospective strand: looking back at the reflection

During her reflection, Elizabeth had felt that it was inappropriate at that time to look at a programme with Ann. Ann was too upset and it was decided that she should make another time to see her when the distress was not so great. She felt that that was the right course to take, and I concurred. We therefore looked at some of the underlying issues.

The substratum strand: the 'messy mirror'

When I asked Elizabeth how she felt about the interview, she became very subdued and looked down at the floor. When I asked her what had happened, she stated that she had found Ann's tears very uncomfortable and had felt helpless to know what to do, and so had left the interview earlier than she might have done, with an excuse that she had to see another patient. She felt very bad about doing so, partly because she had not felt able to comfort Ann in any way, and also because she felt that she should have handled the situation differently. At that point she asked for some time to go and think about the events, as she felt her head was too 'muddled'.

The connective strand: making sense of the image

When we met again, Elizabeth was initially very apprehensive at talking. She started to avoid eye contact, and fidgeted in her chair. When I asked her what was troubling her, she started by saying:

> 'I don't want this to count against me, as I'm sure you'll think I'm being really stupid here...'

At that particular point in time I felt that Elizabeth and I had reached a good working relationship and level of understanding, and suggested that she tell me what was happening. So she continued:

> 'When I took time away from the situation, one of the things that struck me was that not only was I uncomfortable in dealing with Ann's tears, but I felt extremely angry with her over her outburst of emotion: it seemed really self-indulgent. As I thought more about my reaction, what it triggered off for me was my own mother's death, and my reactions to it at the time. I was in my twenties and had not had a good relationship with my mum for a long time. I was abroad when she died, having not lived at home for years, and came back the day before the funeral. I can remember not crying at the graveside, and going back abroad a few

days later, and just carrying on with life. I know it sounds strange, but I never really mourned her properly, and hearing Ann talking about her own mother and how much she missed her filled me with all sorts of feelings I would rather not feel.'

She finished with a sigh of relief, and looked me straight in the eye. One of the things that struck me was her honesty in being able to tell me something that was clearly painful to her, and I fed that back to her. We then tried to summarise the issues, as we saw them. We came up with the following list:

- Elizabeth's own distress at interviewing Ann
- The emotions that it had aroused in her
- Her handling of the interview, when she had left early and in what she now appreciated was an unsatisfactory way
- Ann's own treatment needs

The connective strand: the true image reflected back

Elizabeth felt that that was an accurate summary, and so we looked together at how we might tackle each of the issues.

Elizabeth's distress

Although feeling initially apprehensive of telling me, Elizabeth expressed relief that she had managed to do so. However, she also confided the following:

'Many other students are really afraid to tell their supervisors if they're really upset about something, for fear it'll be held against them some- how ... you know ... being seen as weak or not capable. Grades are important, and often there's a fear that the supervisor'll mark them down if they're seen as not coping.'

Together, we looked at the reality about this in terms of whether Elizabeth had coped as badly as she thought. She could have not told me about the underlying reason for her leaving the interview early, and carried on as though nothing had happened. Instead she had chosen to take a risk in telling me, and also expressed her fears about how I might interpret her actions. There was also an issue about what help Elizabeth felt she needed to deal with her own distress and where the most appropriate place and person to deal with it were to be found. She did not feel that it should interfere with the placement, but also felt that she needed to talk to someone and so decided to contact the student counselling service as a preliminary step.

Unfinished business – the interview

Elizabeth felt unhappy about the way in which she had left the interview with Ann, but struggled with knowing how to rectify the situation. Her dilemma was about how much of her own situation she should disclose to Ann in relation to their last conversation, if at all. For her it brought up the issue of therapeutic engagement: how much personal disclosure is it helpful for a patient to know? Elizabeth felt that it was important that she acknowledge Ann's distress, and apologise for failing to do so at the original interview. She was also aware of not making Ann feel guilty about expressing emotion. We looked at what she might say. It went something like this:

'I would like to apologise for rushing away the other day; I feel that I didn't acknowledge the way you were feeling and I am sorry for that. My mother died too, and there are times I feel very emotional about her death.'

Elizabeth did go back to see Ann and tell her the above. She found Ann still distressed but grateful for an explanation as to Elizabeth's sudden disappearance. She had in fact felt that she had said something wrong. She was relieved to know that it was not 'her fault'.

Ann's treatment needs

Elizabeth's dilemma was also that she had let her own emotional agenda get in the way of Ann's needs. Should Elizabeth be the one to carry on working with her, should she withdraw, should we work together? Looking at the options, Elizabeth felt that now she had acknowledged the issue for herself. It was easier to see how she had been blocking treatment. However, she felt that to be the primary Occupational Therapist (OT) involved was not the most helpful solution for Ann. Elizabeth felt that she needed support from me as her supervisor to co-work, as she felt she was too emotionally vulnerable to deal with Ann's issues about bereavement and loss.

I felt that this showed a degree of insight into her own mental health needs. We agreed an arrangement by which we co-worked with Ann. This would not remove her from Ann's gaze and would not lead Ann to feel guilty that her emotions were too much for Elizabeth to deal with. Although Elizabeth did find sessions with Ann difficult in terms of hearing about Ann's losses, she at least was able to acknowledge this in supervision. She got herself some counselling support from outside the situation and we looked constructively when in supervision at how she could protect herself emotionally, while still working in a therapeutic way with Ann and with other patients in the day programme activities. At the end of her placement, Elizabeth shared some of her reflections on the whole incident:

'You know, at the beginning, this was really hard for me [the situation with Ann]...I feel I would have done everything to avoid it but I knew that I couldn't, for her sake as much as mine. The whole incident brought up some really painful memories for me, and I know that it will take some time to come to terms with them. I also know that there will be other Anns out there whom I will meet on placement, and I need to be able to work with them in a constructive way and not let my own mess muddy the issue. It was a 'messy mirror': for a while I couldn't see my own reflection clearly, but I'm glad I didn't rush away from it. When I look back, the reflection is a lot clearer and it's much easier to gaze in and see what the reality is.'

References

Fish, D., Twinn, S. & Purr, B. (1990) *Promoting reflection: Improving the supervision of practice in health visiting and initial teacher training: how to enable students to learn through professional practice.* Report Number 2, West London Institute of Higher Education, London.

Schwartzberg, S. (1993) The therapeutic use of self. In *Willard and Spackman's Occupational Therapy*, 8th edn. Lippincott, Philadelphia.

3.6   CHALLENGING SAM, AN UNDERGRADUATE RADIOGRAPHIC STUDENT

Krysia Lewandowski

Sam is an undergraduate radiographer who has just completed his first year of a three-year training course in diagnostic radiography. He commenced training immediately after completion of his 'A' level courses. He belongs to a strong religious group and admits that he has had few dealings with the general public or with people other than those within his group. At the interview prior to acceptance on the course it was readily noted by the panel that he had an apparent lack of interpersonal skills and minimal experience in short-term encounters. This might raise issues with regard to the development of effective rapport and successful examinations when dealing with staff and patients in a diagnostic-imaging department. Sam himself expressed these concerns himself at his interview. However, he also presented as an academically competent and enthusiastic prospective student and was accepted on to the course.

Good communication is fundamental to the provision of effective health care. In recent years there has been a noteworthy increase in the appreciation of the importance of the interpersonal dimension of the work of health care personnel and the benefits of its contribution to patient well-being, as discussed by Dickson *et al.* (1989, p. 4). Ellis & Whittington (1981, cited in Dickson *et al.* 1989, p.4) regard the health professions collectively as the 'interpersonal professions'. There is much evidence to suggest that interpersonal proficiency is essential to gain trust, mutual understanding, diagnostic efficiency, accurate information and at least, effective management and care (Rogers 1983; Jaques 1984; Ellis 1988; Dickson *et al.* 1989; Evans *et al.* 1991). The skilled social performer can elicit desired responses from those with whom he interacts. A health care professional whose role is concerned mainly with dealing with people, gaining their trust and co-operation and ultimately a certain reaction, has an essential need for an adept social performance (Argyle 1994). With these factors in mind Sam was to be monitored closely with regard to his communication skills using the Oxford Centre for Radiographic Studies (OCRS) clinical competence profile as a tool for measuring progress.

Following completion of his first academic block of 11 weeks, Sam proved himself indeed to be an excellent student academically, although his participation in the modules and exercises designed to reinforce and enhance students' existing communication skills proved to be minimal. Davies & Farmer (1992) point out that those trainees with the weakest skills are often the ones initially most threatened by small group settings. This endorses Argyle's comments about the influence of social and cultural values on personal behaviour and interpersonal skills, and non-verbal means of communication, as well as the rules governing behaviour in different situations (Argyle 1994, p. 166). The student group and the unfamiliar environment as perceived by Sam created a barrier to effective interaction. Davies & Farmer suggest that participants such as Sam are often the ones who develop most rapidly, provided the group has a skilled leader who can ensure that the group remains supportive and non-threatening. The following 12 weeks of Sam's programme would enable him to demonstrate his interpersonal skills.

The first clinical placement to which Sam was allocated was a 'wide-spread imaging' department within a large hospital some miles from the school of radiography. A shift system for staff was in operation, which made it difficult to roster Sam with a particular member of staff for any significant length of time. It was therefore awkward to monitor his interactions with colleagues and patients. As his designated mentor visiting the department only once a week and with four other students to see in the same department, I had very little time to observe his progress closely. Since I had very little time I had to gain most of my information and to develop my opinions through discussions with Sam himself, the clinical staff of the department, his peers and Sam's end of placement reports. The conclusion drawn by senior clinical staff at the end of this placement was that Sam did have a communication difficulty. Staff had attempted to involve him in their conversations and had encouraged him to undertake examinations unassisted to practise his communication skills. Slight progress had been made but his clinical competence profile indicated that he was below the minimum level expected for a student at his stage of training.

Following this placement I had a discussion with Sam. It then became evident that the department was in fact large enough for the student to 'lose himself', and an accurate assessment of his needs had not been made. However, during this discussion, I felt that our relationship as mentor/mentee entered the *initiation* stage. Morton-Cooper & Palmer (1993) describe the start or initiation of a relationship as being the 'locking on' of individuals, the 'getting to know you' period. Many analyses of the role of mentor exist and what seems to be common to most of them is the fact that there is always a recognisable start, a developmental stage and then a termination to the relationship (Hunt & Michael 1983; Campbell-Header 1986; Hawkin & Thibodeau 1989 (all cited in Morton-Cooper & Palmer 1993); Darling 1984; Rankin 1991).

The second clinical placement area Sam was to attend was by contrast in a much smaller, more compact department. As a result the difficulties encountered by Sam were very quickly noticed. It became apparent that Sam was withdrawing from the issue rather than facing up to it. Within weeks of starting his placement I was aware of an unfortunate predicament. Sam was becoming a talking point in the staff room. Eraut suggests that learning is either facilitated or constrained by the social climate of the work environment (Eraut 1998). The informal role of those working alongside a learner is probably more important than their formal role. Sam was becoming labelled as lazy, disinterested and 'stand-offish'. His lack of interpersonal skills was the subject of ridicule and the opportunities for him to learn from the clinical placement were becoming severely impeded. I felt it was essential to tackle the situation immediately and directly. I arranged to spend a day working alongside Sam in the clinical environment; our relationship was entering a new phase, the *working* or training phase. This is where the main focus for individual growth and development lies. The dynamics of the mentoring relationship are maintained by the joint interaction of both individuals and the increasing trust and closeness that begin to develop (Morton-Cooper & Palmer 1993, p. 71).

During our conversation following the clinical session, Sam told me how very discouraged and disheartened he was feeling. He was aware of his inadequacy in communicating with peers, colleagues and patients, and through his learning contract he indicated that he had very few thoughts on how to alleviate the problem. (On this course a learning contract is a document drawn up by the undergraduate student to identify and achieve personal goals. It includes identification of the resources that might be available.) Sam appeared to be oblivious to the severity of the situation or to the fact that he was becoming a laughing stock. In order to resolve this predicament the situation had to be clearly identified and so problem solving of the type advocated by Gibbs *et al.* (1988) was initiated (see Fig. 3.1).

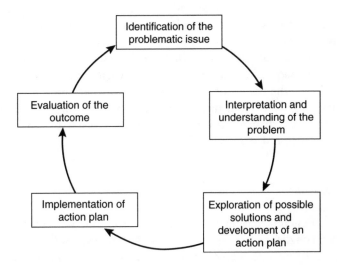

Fig. 3.1. A problem-solving cycle.

Sam was very embarrassed, anxious and then concerned as I disclosed the situation as perceived by others. Together we aimed to establish the extent and source of the problems and issues raised within their associated frames of reference. I was aware of my distinct need to handle the situation skilfully in order to produce the desired effect. This was to persuade Sam to learn that I was his ally and facilitator. My concern was to prevent any notions of inadequacy and hopelessness. In progressing through the stages depicted by the problem-solving cycle, a number of solutions were discussed and we began to feel that a strong mentoring relationship was beginning to develop rapidly. This reflects findings described by Morton-Cooper & Palmer (1993) in their research and depends upon openness and close collaboration between the student and the mentor thus creating a climate of mutual trust and sharing.

My next visit to the department was a highly satisfactory one. Many comments were made concerning the great improvement evident in Sam's attitude and approach to both staff and patients. The fact that he had made a particular effort in using suggestions that I had made, such as to become involved in conversations, reassured me that my mentorship had successfully helped Sam's personal and professional development. He was beginning to disclose something of his own opinions, thus becoming not only more receptive but also more of an initiator. As a result, social encounters became far more enjoyable for Sam, and as staff began to relate to his personality and character rather than to his inability his learning environment became more potent. The nature of his communication process was becoming more transactional rather than linear. Early theorists considered communication as a linear process, but more recently the process has come to be viewed as a transactional activity which is influenced by the reception and the responses made by the participants in the act of talking to each other (Dickson *et al.* 1989). In Sam's case not only had he become more involved when talking to patients and colleagues, but the nature of his interactions was becoming active rather than passive. Clinical staff quickly became aware of the effort Sam was making to strengthen his social skills and as a result his environment became happier and more supportive.

Conclusion

In this particular situation I felt it was appropriate and essential to be direct or to challenge Sam by being open and honest and by making him fully aware of the difficulties that he was creating in his clinical environment. It was a difficult decision for me to make as such a confrontational and challenging stance could easily have had a detrimental effect. This could have increased the likelihood of Sam feeling frustrated and isolated. I simply reminded him of some shortcomings over which he had little control. By contrast, to have sheltered him from the truth would not have provided the opportunities for growth. This was a risk that I felt that I had to take. Sam had already demonstrated an immaturity in handling the situation when he tried to resolve it. (In using the term 'immaturity', I apply it in a positive manner as expressed by Dewey (1916/1966) and see it not as a lack or absence of powers but as a positive force – the ability to develop, the power to grow.

As a result of my willingness to take the risk and my openness, Sam gained confidence and with this a degree of independence to try out his own ideas, comfortable in the knowledge that I could be trusted to support and guide him if necessary. This reflected the strength of our relationship and the degree of trust that we were able to develop. The situation encountered by Sam bears a strong resemblance to the process described by Taylor (1987), which I have illustrated with descriptions of Sam's progress.

- **Disconfirmation** – Sam was aware of the problem; it caused anxiety and confusion and a wish to withdraw from the experiences causing the conflict.
- **Exploration** – We explored the problem in an open and collaborative way. This made it possible for Sam to gain insight, confidence and some satisfaction.
- **Reflection** – Through discussions with me and by writing up his experiences in his personal diary Sam was able to develop a new approach to his learning task.
- **Sharing the discovery** – Trying out his new thinking was a positive experience and we both shared in the satisfaction of seeing the progress he made.

The final phase of *equilibrium* will hopefully be demonstrated in time. Taylor's framework highlights the difficult and frustrating phases that can take place in many learning experiences. In this case study I hope I have demonstrated the need for a supportive mentor who is able to provide emotional encouragement, to instil confidence and to foster risk-taking. An American nurse in 1984 defined three basic mentoring roles: inspirer, investor and supporter (Darling 1984). In my experience, realisation of these roles can only take place when both the student and the mentor have made a commitment and when a trusting relationship exists between them. The role of mentor is not an easy one to play but it can give great satisfaction when the role is valued and functional.

Epilogue

Sam successfully completed his training as a diagnostic radiographer. He secured employment in a large teaching hospital and has since gained a wealth of experience and insight. His skills have enabled him to work abroad also. He is still softly spoken and a placid member of his peer group. However, he now demonstrates a purposefulness, a quiet confidence and a sense of humour which at one time would not have been considered possible. The mentoring relationship has long since diminished but Sam has kept in touch, letting me know how his career and life are progressing and occasionally turning to me for an opportunity to discuss his next step. As his one-time mentor it is immensely satisfying to know that I was able to provide guidance and strength to mobilise his skills and that he feels able to return to that alliance at times; an effective mentoring relationship provides mutual professional development and fulfilment.

References

Argyle, M. (1994) *The Psychology of Interpersonal Behaviour,* 5th edn. Penguin Books, London.

Campbell-Header, N. (1986) Do nurses need mentors? *Image: Journal of Nursing Scholarship* **18** (3), 110–13.

Darling, L.A.W. (1984) The mentoring dimension. What do nurses want in a mentor? *Journal of Nursing Administration* October, 42–4.

Davies, P.G. & Farmer, E. A. (1992) Teaching communication skills in small groups. *Medical Journal of Australia* 56, February.

Dewey, J. (1916/1966) *Democracy and Education.* Free Press, New York.

Dickson, D. A., Hargie, O. & Morrow, N. C. (1989) *Communication Skills Training for Health Professionals: An Instructor's Handbook.* Chapman & Hall, London.

Ellis, R. (1988) *Professional Competence and Quality Assurance in the Caring Professions.* Chapman & Hall, London.

Eraut, M. (1988) Learning in the workplace. *Training Officer* **34** (6), 172–4.

Evans, B. J., Stanley, R. O., Mestrovic, R. & Rose, L. (1991) Effects of communication skills training on students' diagnostic efficiency. *Medical Education* **25**, 517–26.

Gibbs, G., Habershaw, S. & Habershaw, T. (1988) *53 Interesting Ways to Appraise Your Teaching.* Technical and Educational Services Ltd, Bristol.

Hawkins, J.W. & Thibodeau, J.A. (1989) *The Nurse Practitioner and Clinical Nurse Specialist. Current Practice Issues,* 2nd edn. Tiresias Press, New York.

Hunt, D. & Michael, C. (1983) Mentorship: a career training in development tool. *Academy of Management Review* 3 475–85.

Jaques, D. (1984) *Learning in Groups.* Croom Helm, London.

Morton-Cooper A. & Palmer, A. (1993) *Mentoring and Preceptorship: A Guide to Support Roles in Clinical Practice.* Blackwell Science, Oxford.

Rankin, E. A. D. (1991) Mentor, mentee, mentoring: building career development relationships. *Nursing Connections* 4 (4), 49–51.

Rogers, R. (1983) *Freedom to Learn for the 80s.* Charles E. Merrill, New York.

Taylor, M. (1987) Self-directed learning: more than meets the observer's eye. In *Appreciating Adults Learning: From the Learners' Perspective* (D. Boud & V. Griffin, eds), pp. 179–96. Kogan Page, London.

3.7 LEARNING TO PROMOTE PERSONAL PROFESSIONAL PRACTICE

Claire-Louise Hatton

In this critical incident I shall explore an issue concerning the extent of a clinical supervisor's role in promoting professional practice. The incident arose following a clinical supervision session with one of my students who is learning to be a traditional acupuncturist. I was disappointed about the way in which this student, whom I shall call Phil, was developing and whilst anticipating a tutorial session I was prompted to reflect on my feelings. My role is both college- and profession-based (Fish *et al.* 1990). To reflect on the incident and to support my analysis I will use the work of the nursing theorist Barbara Carper (1978). Carper identifies four fundamental patterns of 'knowing' in nursing knowledge: empirical, aesthetic, personal knowledge and moral knowledge. She argues that each aspect of knowledge is necessary but not complete alone to validate an approach to learning within a discipline. As a clinical supervisor for Year three student-practitioners my responsibilities include:

- Supervising the treatment of patients
- Personal tutoring of students in respect of their acupuncture studies
- Continuous assessment of individual students' work and development
- Being available for support, consultations, supervisions or phone-line help

In this role the tutorial aspects are primarily to do with course-related issues. The third year is a transitional stage in the course and some student-practitioners are honest about finding difficulty with this change from supervised practice to independent work. As a clinical supervisor, one of the difficulties is to gauge what level and what kind of support a student practitioner needs. As a supervisor in the teaching clinic I am able to form impressions of and insights into students as they practise on patients. Intuitive knowledge can be invaluable and is particularly important with patients. But such knowledge needs to be validated.

Insights about students do not always have a tidy place to go, neither can they be useful in assessment and they drift unsatisfactorily in one's consciousness. Someone can fulfil all the requirements, be proficient, professional and yet... What is one's moral, rather than contractual, obligation within the description of the role of supervisor to provide feedback? This is the nub of the question that I needed to explore.

The student-practitioners

The student-practitioners with whom I was concerned were in the final six months of their three-year programme. In Year three, professional development and clinical reasoning are monitored closely through case notes (these are submitted for all treatments carried out) and students' portfolio work, which is the primary means of assessment at this stage. The onus is on the student to ask for any additional support in between visits to college. Tutorials are scheduled and there is informal contact on visits. In their portfolio, students are expected to document continuing professional development through self-appraisal and critical reflection. This should include using a reflective learning cycle to record their experiences and critical incidents, and to develop self-awareness of their personal beliefs, values and personal communication style as they impact upon their work with patients. The hope is that as a result of their exploration and discussion within supervision, student-practitioners will develop a clearer sense of the clinical choices available to them. They should be better able to validate their treatment approaches, and have sufficient resources for help and self-development. I feel that there is an element of tension when fulfilling my dual role as supervisor, where I contribute to students' assessment whilst also working alongside them with patients. This role includes the exploration of clinical approaches and reasoning while also trying to model professional artistry (Schön 1987). The approach embraces uncertainty and is informed by a philosophy that practice is not just a series of tasks but an activity which is informed by awareness of values and which acknowledges that theory emerges from practice.

The critical incident

On this particular occasion I had spent the morning acting as clinical supervisor to two students whom I have called David and Phil. Both had brought patients to the treatment clinic for one-off supervision to fulfil a final requirement of their programme. By this stage students are expected to present a full diagnosis with sound clinical reasoning for their treatment strategy. Before, during and after seeing the patients we discussed their treatment strategies and issues arising from treatment, both clinically and for themselves. The session had proceeded without any major difficulty. I was thinking about the session and considering the approach I would take in the personal tutoring session with each student that afternoon. I became aware that my dominant feelings were dissatisfaction and frustration with my role as tutor resulting in a sense of 'heart-sink' at the prospect of the forthcoming session with Phil. This, I realised, was not an isolated occurrence but a frequent sense of disquiet about not having served a student as well as I might. Acknowledging these feelings and their frequency made me wish to investigate further. Tripp (1993) identifies that the vast majority of critical incidents are accounts of very commonplace events that occur in professional practice. Such events become critical in the sense that they are indicative of underlying trends, motives and structures. It is only through analysing such events that they become critical. Both Phil and David behaved in ways consistent with my previous experience of them. What I found disappointing was the limited approach Phil was taking to develop himself as a practitioner. The programme emphasises ongoing professional development and inquiry into practice as inextricably linked with self-development. The course curriculum is based on a belief that the spirit of inquiry needed for professional development also affects evaluation of personal values (College of Traditional Acupuncture 1998).

Process-oriented professional development

David

Of the two students, David was the one in whom I saw changes which made me believe that I had fulfilled my role and facilitated his development in such a way that he was better equipped, more resourceful and independent than he was at the start of the clinical supervision period. What seemed different with David was mostly his professional development work. David and Phil were at an identical point in their course. Up to this point both had fulfilled their assessments and met their learning intentions. Their personalities and educational profiles were obviously very different. I came to see that this played a part in why I didn't serve each equally well. What, I wondered, made the supervision with David seemingly more successful? He was an anxious, retiring person but managed to make good use of the telephone support offered and was able to ask for help when needed. Although he felt less confident about theoretical aspects of the material than some students, he recognised that the real problem was that of confidence. We had discussed strategies and addressed aspects causing him any particular loss of confidence. It wasn't that as a tutor I was able or wanting to fix the problem. It was more a situation where the openness, emotional honesty and flexibility of David responding to my genuine interest made the work of tutoring become alive. I wasn't in the position of the one with more answers, or the one there to judge but a resource for him to talk things through to some further clarity. Massarik (1979) identifies six styles of interview: the hostile; the limited survey; rapport; asymmetrical trust; depth and phenomenal. David and I worked at the depth interview level where the interviewer explores thoroughly the views and dynamics of the interviewee who reciprocates and responds in appropriate depth. More importantly in the long run was the fact that David, unlike Phil, had managed to really engage with and use the entire reflective learning cycle. His portfolio work showed awareness and meaningful insight into his process, coupled with the development and evaluation of action plans. He uncovered connections and patterns in his work, both theoretically and personally. He had a critical edge with a real spirit of inquiry. It was this that made me feel more hopeful about his future professional development. He had resources for investigating his practice, which he was familiar with and regarded as worthwhile. Tutoring sessions, while not always easy, were stimulating and rewarding rather than formal and awkward.

Phil

Phil had been working with two patients that morning. One was very ill and both had complicated diagnoses. Phil's work was diagnostically and technically excellent. But his treatment rationale lacked exploration of the patients' needs, and discussion revealed he had not looked at his own process and responses to treating in these difficult circumstances. Phil was very bright and meticulous, and gave the impression of being extremely competent. He never asked for any additional support. His reflective pieces in his portfolio never probed beyond obligation and were as short as possible. In previous tutorials I would try to elicit evidence of his internal process and he would respond with ready answers and textbook rationales for treatment. He was a relatively young student. I felt he compensated for his lack of life experiences and the value given to these on the course by being well versed in all theory, indeed impressively so. In some ways he was unwilling or unable to show his vulnerability and uncertainty, and somewhat defensive when challenged. Other programme requirements were met promptly and his practice size increased satisfactorily. In his self-development work he was always chasing deadlines and never implemented any of the agreed courses of action to remedy this. Phil's work was more strategic than David's.

The value of reflective portfolio work increases as students commit themselves to the process. They begin to perceive its usefulness and relevance not just to their work but to their life. This was not evidenced by Phil. Given the high quality of his work overall I found it hard to justify pursuing further exchanges or requirements and was left with a sense that his professional exterior was guarding some insecurity that I as tutor had not garnered enough trust to penetrate. It was too easy to accept what was offered rather than confront what was missing. Ultimately this was disappointing, as I believe it robbed the exchange of richness and lost what could have been interesting explorations of values with a good student. I imagine that the comfort zone of development for this student was never challenged sufficiently or specifically. A veneer of professionalism displaced his discomfort about his inexperience. Although I intended to work at the level of Massarik's depth interview and genuinely to explore Phil's process, I felt distanced by his defensiveness and reluctance to explore his responses more deeply. So we operated at best at the level of the rapport interview where 'the "door" is opened to a more genuinely human relationship between interview and interviewee' (Massarik 1979). In this situation there is some deeper interpersonal contact between participants but the process is strictly confined, although with regard to some of the content Phil's responses fell more into that of the limited survey interview where he made little effort to actively participate in the discussion. How could I shift the level of the exchange to one that was more meaningful and in accord with the value of professional self-development? Interestingly, David was not necessarily the better or more intelligent student of the two. By implication there was some aspect of the process-orientated professional development work as evidenced through his portfolio that Phil was not addressing. Phil was completing the programme requirements but other, less definable aspects that come into professional development were not undertaken as fully as was expected.

There is a fine line between what is tangible and possible to evidence and what is intangible and discernible through subjective observation or intuition about a person. These less tangible aspects of a curriculum, which are part of practitioner development, can sometimes be adhered to in letter rather than in spirit. Students who are not truly reflective can still become adept at providing sufficient evidence to meet learning intentions, or can do so at a much more superficial level than they might (Gibbs 1992). I realised that it was too easy to say it was simply a matter of personality, which would appear to blame the student or some dynamic between student and supervisor. I do not believe a professional learning outcome can be based on something as random as this.

Questions

Were the students clear as to the course requirements?

> Yes, I had checked and discussed these with them at their previous session, and they were also made clear in their handbook. In discussion they showed an understanding of the rationale for this teaching style. However, I believe that when students do not experience process-based learning in school, it can take a long time for them to adapt to a process-based education. The level of sophistication required by the programme had not proved too onerous for most students.

Had enough time been scheduled to explore what was to be gained through portfolio work?

> The values of a course need to be not only explicit but thoroughly explored. Given that students did know what the requirements were, I thought along other lines.

Were these less tangible requirements actually necessary? After all, if they could work safely and provide good clinical reasoning, should an institution say that students must adhere to this model? Was this not just an ideal, one that is not realisable in all cases?

> Well, perhaps, except that as a profession that espouses the value of lifelong learning and on-going practitioner development, it seems important that habits of reflective learning are encouraged early. Otherwise some practitioners will never evaluate their practice, will never articulate and know what they do know and what they don't know. Neither will they necessarily have a strategy for professional development. Recognising and applying the value of active reflection, reflection-in-action and general research-mindedness keeps practice alive and challenging. It avoids working solely from habit and is vital when one is working with individuals.

If a profession is truly seen as a 'body of individuals', then it is important that each part of that body, each individual, knows what they are contributing as well as what they agree to uphold.

Shu Ha Ri

If one accepts Carper's position that each of the four patterns of knowing are important yet insufficient alone, and professional artistry is something practitioners aspire to and consider a value, then, yes, there is an obligation to assist someone towards their self-knowledge. Reflection refines and deepens our authenticity through which one 'finds and possesses oneself' (Larre *et al.* 1995). It develops acuity of perception and compassion as well as the 'consciousness of possibilities' (Kaptchuk 1992, Communication). Professional artistry combines skill, reflection and practice blended to become recognisably our own personal style. It moves beyond fact and encapsulates what we learn initially woven through with individual experience, research and choices made. There is a Japanese term, Shu Ha Ri, which arose originally from the Japanese tea ceremony and continues as a traditional teaching method, meaning:

'What we absorb and obey, we must eventually break away from. To merely follow our teacher's tradition is not sufficient but it is a necessary starting point. You must develop your sensitivity and allow your intuition to develop. If you can open your senses and your mind, you will learn to see the subtle nuances of each patient's condition ... you will slowly master treatment and develop your own treatment style.' (Manaka *et al.* 1995)

In a similar vein Carper (1978) uses the work of Wiedenbach (1964) to describe the artistry of nursing. In doing so she argues that:

'The art of nursing is made visible through the action taken to provide whatever the patient requires to restore or extend his ability to cope with the demands of his situation.'

To have an aesthetic quality the action taken requires:

'The active transformation of the immediate object – the patient behaviour – into a direct, non mediated perception of what is significant in it – that is, what need is actually being expressed by the behaviour. The perception of the need expressed is not only responsible for the action taken by the nurse but reflected in it.'

Carper goes on to say that empathy is important in the aesthetic pattern of knowing. This, together with personal knowledge, is described by Carper as:

'the knowing, encountering and actualising of the concrete, individual self ... which is ... standing in relation to another human being as a person ... as well as [taking] the risk of commitment. (Carper 1978, p. 17)

It has to be recognised that to be a health professional not only involves the carrying out of tasks but also involves character and awareness of morals. This is evident in the fact that professions have codes of conduct. Moral choices involve knowledge of oneself and of one's own values. The relationship of practitioner and patient has much in common with that between tutor and student-practitioner. Could I ask this student to risk his sense of safety in self-exploration, the better to meet the particular needs of his patients, if I would not take that risk with him? Previously, both students had been encouraged verbally and in writing to specify what would be useful to them in terms of feedback, support, etc. David had taken this up alone. So what was stopping Phil? This was the puzzle. What could I do differently?

Action

I felt there was a case for sharing my puzzlement, impressions and intuitions with Phil, although this went beyond my role as specified. The dilemma was to find a way to discuss these observations with Phil without alienating him. Honesty concerning issues the student may not want to discuss or may not be open to hearing can be difficult, especially if there are no factual criteria to consolidate one's observations. The challenge was about the courage to comment, to be sure that what I had in mind truly was in the best interest of the student. It highlighted the tensions inherent in the role and the moral dimensions of supervision. I wanted to find a way to offer my observations in the hope that our discussion could be more real and the learning edge more fruitful. I felt anxious about doing so, but I believed that until I put forward my observations, whilst acknowledging their subjectivity, the interaction would not be authentic. Going beyond the strict definition of my role as supervisor, which in many ways I had been happy with, made me uncomfortable. I am not trained as a counsellor and while through staff development one learns appropriate forms of giving feedback, I preferred to keep my observations work-related. However, here I felt impelled to offer my observations. Otherwise I would feel I had allowed something to slip by without dealing with it and the discussion would remain superficial for the sake of a moment of discomfort.

Phil consented to receive feedback of this nature. With Phil, until I addressed the issue of his impenetrable veneer of professionalism, nothing felt real. He was defensive, claiming to have fulfilled all that had been required of him but did volunteer that to be 'real' and to work collaboratively rather than competitively was very uncomfortable and he could not see a way to change this. He did not feel he could access his own process and was not convinced that this was worthwhile anyway as he saw professionalism as doing things well and abiding by the code of conduct. Theory fascinated him but he didn't see why he should look at his development in this context. I viewed this as at least having opened a door to future exchange and exploration, and felt that I had said what I felt obliged to say.

I thought it was worthwhile giving my observations. In future this aspect could be made explicit within my role from the beginning with each student. Students know from their assessment criteria that their development will be commented upon. I had taken refuge within the strict definition of my role to evade aspects that I found uncomfortable. I do not see that it will necessarily result in any earth-shattering insights. But it will allow me to see congruence between the values held by the programme and my own actions. This experience confirmed that there is a place for personal comment and observation. I had the experience that this doesn't have to be uncomfortably personal or confronting. Although it may be challenging it can also be creative, provided it is owned, and this has encouraged me to continue. It seems sensible, given the subjective nature of impressions, to discuss (within the boundaries of confidentiality) my observations with a colleague beforehand to see if the problem is merely my own. It has made me more aware of the tensions between the role of supervisor who has some input into assessment and trying to model a process-based programme. It remains a challenge to convey the full potential of reflective learning and to convey the value and relevance of different types of knowledge within professional artistry to the work of a practitioner.

References

Carper, B. A. (1978) Fundamental patterns of knowing in nursing. *Advances in Nursing Science* 1, 13–23.

College of Traditional Acupuncture (1998) *Definitive Document*. CTA, Leamington Spa.

Fish, D., Twinn, S. & Purr, B. (1990) Promoting reflection: improving the supervision of practice in health visiting and initial teacher training: how to enable students to learn through professional practice. Report Number 2, West London Institute of Higher Education, London.

Gibbs, G. (1992) *Improving the Quality of Student Learning*. Technical and Educational Services, Bristol.

Larre, C. & Rochat de la Vallée, E. (1995) *Rooted in Spirit: The Heart of Chinese Medicine. A Sinological Interpretation of Chapter Eight of Huangdi Neijing Lingshu*. Station Hill Press, New York.

Manaka, Y., Itaya, K. & Birch, S. (1995) *Chasing the Dragon's Tail*. Paradigm Publications, Brookline, Massachusetts.

Massarik, F. (1979) The interviewing process re-examined. In *Human Inquiry: A Sourcebook of New Paradigm Research* (P. Reason & J. Rowan, eds), pp. 201–6. John Wiley, Chichester.

Schön, D. (1987) *Educating the Reflective Practitioner*. Jossey Bass, London.

Tripp, D. (1993) *Critical Incidents in Teaching*. Routledge, London.

Wiedenbach, E. (1964) *Clinical Nursing: A Helping Art*. Springer, New York.

3.8   IMPROVING THE ABILITY TO LEARN FROM EXPERIENCE IN CLINICAL SETTINGS

Louise Dumas

Society today expects health professionals to be autonomous in their thinking and their achievements, to solve professional problems adequately and rapidly, to adapt swiftly and creatively to changes in their environments, and to work continuously towards self-actualisation. Society also requires them to be autonomous and accountable, to transfer easily their knowledge from one domain to another, and to be committed and efficient in very complex situations (Dumas 1995, 1997a). In order to achieve such long-range professional goals, health professionals need to learn how to reflect on their own experience in order to learn from it and to transfer this intimate knowledge into other situations requiring the same type of learning (Burnard 1983; Dumas 1995). However, where and how to learn such abilities remains problematic.

For example, some Canadian universities offer post-diploma baccalaureate programmes to nurses. Those students are adults who have accumulated life and professional experiences which they often don't use in their actual practice, at least not consciously. This has prompted some faculty members to focus their teaching efforts towards strategies which facilitate reflection on one's professional practice, as suggested for example by Brookfield (1987) in education, Deane & Campbell (1985) and Burnard (1991) in nursing, and Etienne (1991) in occupational therapy.

Dumas (1995) elaborated and validated an instrument to help supervisors evaluate the experiential learning of nurse–students during an intensive practicum in clinical settings. First designed as a tool for the supervisors, it has been used since by both supervisors and students as one way to reflect on experiences as they are encountered during the practicum. The Dumas tool was developed for a typical practicum in the post-RN baccalaureate programme; the latter is designed for nurses who graduated from a professional nursing school and wished to pursue studies at university level. The Dumas tool was so appreciated by these students as an aid in their thinking process that they then used it in their daily practice as professionals. Some experiences of this type of reflection during a clinical practicum have prompted professional growth not only for adult students but also for their supervisors and their university professor.

Critical incident

Mary is 30 years old and she has been a full-time nurse on an adult surgical ward in a general hospital for the last 8 years. She is usually recognised as a 'good nurse' by both her colleagues and her superiors, and she is aware of it. Last year, she enrolled part-time in a post-RN baccalaureate programme at the nearby university; she expects this degree will help her to eventually get a job as assistant head nurse or clinical leader on her unit. Up to now, Mary has been able to adequately share her time between her husband, her three-year-old son, her friends, her job, and her studies, but she has to be really organised to get such good results. She is now in the middle of the first practicum of this particular programme (Dumas 1997b). This clinical experience is taking place on her usual working site where she functions with a student's status. She is not involved with patients other than those assigned to her and does not cover other nurses when they are going away from the unit; she also has fewer patients to take care of whether the unit is busy or not. This practicum is two weeks in duration; full time, and pursues the following objectives:

- Apply in real life situations what has been thoroughly studied during the first year, i.e. nursing process based on a nursing theoretical framework, nurse/patient interaction theory
- Reflect on one's own learning from experience in order to begin learning to learn from these experiences

There is a supervisor on site for eight students and her work is to facilitate the attainment of the two objectives for each student. Of course, since the students are already professionals, she does not have to supervise their clinical work on the unit. Her goals are to help students link theory to practice and facilitate their experiential learning. The supervisor is recruited, educated, and closely supervised by a professor (Manley 1997).

Like all the other students, Mary meets daily with her supervisor, Susan, to reflect on the experiences that are unfolding (Krikorian & Paulanka 1982; Palmer *et al.* 1995). In order to respond to the second objective, she has to complete a diary every night, reflecting on specific questions, and then submit it to the supervisor the next morning (Krikorian & Paulanka 1982; Bennett & Kingham 1993). This constitutes the starting point for the discussion on what is going on during the practicum and how she can enhance her learning from this experience as it is unveiling. Susan also meets with all of her students at the end of the day for a post-clinical day discussion. This allows the group to share experiences of the day and to help each other link theory to practice. They can express concerns, frustrations and positive realisations, as well as plan new experimentations for the next day.

This particular practicum is based on an experiential learning philosophy where the adult students are encouraged to learn how to learn from experience. The questions in the students' diaries and the ones leading the group discussions are focused on this objective of enhancing this particular type of students' learning. The Dumas tool was developed for this purpose since no instrument was available for the supervisors to help the students reflect through their own intimate process of learning while it was unfolding during a practicum. An excerpt from this instrument is appended at the end of the chapter; the tool is based on a model of experiential learning competencies developed by Charbonneau & Chevrier (1990) from the Université du Quebec à Hull (Quebec, Canada) after the works of Kolb (1984). It is made of behaviours identified within five distinct stages of experiential learning how to learn: learning management (LM), concrete experience (CE), reflective observation (RO), abstract conceptualisation (AC), and active experimentation (AE). According to the authors, a person who knows how to learn from her own experience will put in action conducts and abilities in each of those five areas and will know how to use them adequately in order to learn more significantly. When learning from an experience, a person can consciously reflect on this actual process of learning in order to readjust efforts when necessary. The behaviours in the Dumas tool guide the learner into such in-depth reflection on their actual experiences. First designed as a formative evaluation self-standing instrument, it is now preferably used as a framework for questions students answer daily in their logbooks.

On the fourth day of the practicum, Mary admits to Susan that she is fed up with this turning around of ideas; she talks about losing time and money, since she is not paid during that practicum she loses more than the supervisor can imagine, etc. She also complains of not having time to care for the same number of patients she usually does; that this type of experience is not realistic; and that she doesn't understand why she is required to do this since she is already recognised as a good nurse. She finds it is absurd to try to go deeper into what she feels and thinks. She thinks that nurses cannot get time to do that; they just have to function with more and more patients who are sicker than they used to be. She believes she should be granted the university credits without this practicum since she knows all that is needed about the nursing process based on a nursing theoretical framework, and about nurse/patient interactions; the supervisor should not forget that she has been a nurse for 8 years. She finds it childish to be asked to reflect on what she does, feels and thinks every day. She says she knows what she is doing and why and that she doesn't need to tell anyone else, such as her supervisor or her colleagues. Her diary has been reflecting such frustrations for the last two days.

This type of reaction surprises Susan since she sincerely believes the opposite. She finds that her students are very lucky to get time to link theory to practice in their real-life situations, to get to apply all they have learned during the last year and this without being under pressure from their peers and the daily turmoil of work. She decides she has to work with Mary in going deeper into her frustrations and find out where all this comes from. By questioning and raising hesitations, Susan explores Mary's experiences of the week. (The initials in parenthesis denote the category in the Dumas model).

S. Mary, did anything specific happen this morning which makes you feel so unsatisfied? In fact, tell me what happened since I saw you yesterday afternoon. (CE)

M. Nothing unusual, it is always the same thing day after day. I tell you, I have the impression I am only playing with ideas and feelings, and that I don't do anything useful on the unit.

S. Yesterday, you wrote in your diary that you felt it was childish to reflect day after day on what you do. What makes you feel this way? (RO)

M. Well, I have learned everything I know and everything I need to know in nursing school. You know, I have been a nurse for 8 years. Don't tell me I didn't know what I have been doing for the last 8 years.

S. Mary, do you think I doubt your clinical competence? (AC)

M. Well, you always challenge me with your questions. I feel I have to know everything, that I should know more and more, that I should read and be curious about nursing stuff. You know what I mean.

S. Do I hear that when I raise questions during our meeting and during the post-clinical discussions, you feel threatened in your competence? (RO)

M.   Well, yes, I guess this is it. You know everyone here thinks I am a good nurse and up to this practicum I thought I was.

S.   Mary, what makes you think you are not any more? (RO)

M.   I told you. I don't know the answers to all your questions. I feel I have to go back to my books every night when I come back home to find answers that will please you.

S.   Mary, why in the world do you have to find answers that will please me? (RO)

M.   Because I want to have good grades for this practicum, I want to show you I am a good nurse and that I know about all that stuff!

And Mary starts to cry. Susan sits silently besides her and hands her a handkerchief.

M.   You know, my colleagues find it is stupid to go back to the university to learn stuff that won't be useful for my daily practice. They keep taunting me every day during coffee time. What did you learn now? Will you be a better nurse now? Oh! Can you do this without your supervisor? And so on, and so on... I am fed up! I thought I would like this practicum but it is not interesting at all! Every day I feel I know less and less and I am afraid nobody will ever consider me as a good nurse any more since now, I question myself about, everything I do! (CE & RO)

S.   Tell me, Mary, did you ever feel this way some other time in your life? (AC)

M.   Hum... Yes, when I came on this unit right after I graduated I had the impression I did not remember a thing of what I had learned in school and during my clinical experiences. (RO)

S.   And do you remember what you did to feel more comfortable day after day?

M.   I used to look in my books every night and check everything I had not known during the day so I would know the following day.

S.   And you stopped doing it after a while.

M.   Well, yes, since most of the patients come for the same type of diagnosis and same type of surgery I don't have to go in my books any more.

S.   How come you have to go to your books then for this practicum?

M.   Because I started back doubting about me, about my competence you know. Nobody ever asked me so many questions since I started on this unit. But you do!

S.   And it challenges you.

M.   Yes, I feel incompetent again, as when I graduated.

S.   Mary, did you discuss this with the other students in the group?

M.   No.

S.   Can you imagine that everyone may be feeling the same way?

M.   No. It did not even occur to me.

S.   Mary, do you remember we have discussed Benner's work during the class on professional matters? How she comes about with different levels of nursing competence? (AC)

Susan explains the normalcy of this feeling during a practicum with adult students, that they should bring this matter for the afternoon discussion so that everyone could get a chance to express herself on this subject (in order to get to AE).

After a very useful discussion with the group, Susan goes back home. She is upset, anxious and insecure. She wonders if maybe she really is challenging her students too much. She feels she has to call the professor in charge of the practicum, with whom she discusses all of her own insecurities. Louise receives her with warmth and openness. She has been a supervisor herself before and knows how frustrating it can be at times, and how much work it represents. She also recalls what Manley (1997) considers basic effective adult education practice: experience and expertise of the preceptor, understanding and appreciation of learning, warmth, respect, and consistency, uniqueness of the learner's experience, the need for partnership in learning relationships, etc.

Debriefing

Brookfield (1990) describes the profound psychological disruption that often accompanies learning and how frequently people prefer to remain in unsatisfactory situations rather than have to make the necessary adjustments and changes (Brookfield 1990, p.147).

Coming back to the university, adult students often feel challenged by the new learning that takes place. They realise they don't know everything and that coming back to school is not just getting a certificate. In fact, in their daily practice, they also face complex problems that are insoluble by rational technical approach alone, and some nurses then just fall into a daily routine with their patients to avoid what Brookfield calls psychological disruption. Coming back to school to get a degree makes them realise they have to learn and not just be there. Learning involves change and this is challenging, since it requires critical reflection on thoughts and actions that have previously been taken for granted. This also means producing new habits by learning how to think of themselves differently. On the other hand, as preceptors or clinical supervisors, nurses are used to challenging themselves and others in their thinking and their doing, and they may not realise that some students or peers become insecure with this exercise. Because self-esteem as adults and as competent professionals is put at stake, supervisors need to learn how to stimulate students without putting them in such turmoil that change is viewed as a danger.

Both the student and the clinical supervisor need a tool to help them reflect on what they do in their day-to-day practice. Dumas (1995) has developed and validated such a tool. It is congruent with an experiential learning philosophy and one of learning how to learn as a life long process. Thirty-two behaviours have been identified as part of a reflective process that should take place during this type of practicum and also during usual professional nursing practice. These behaviours can be presented as questions to be answered in diaries.

When an event is first experienced in a holistic manner (CE), it produces cognitive, affective, and operational elements that can be reflected upon when the nurse takes the role of an observer of her own experience (RO). From the resulting observations and reflections, she can elaborate some mental schemes (AC) that are very well away from her actual experience but that can be tested against the reality of her nursing practice (AE). Using the behaviours that have been identified in the Dumas tool the supervisor can facilitate this process of critically reflecting on one's own experience. This is what Susan did in order to help Mary reflect on her practicum (see letters in parentheses, corresponding to three of the five phases of the tool). This is also what Louise did to help Susan reflect on her own experience as Mary's supervisor. In fact, what this tool does is to help the assessment of the intimate progression of learning in an individual person. It helps define hidden agendas, motives behind actions or thoughts on a particular experience. The learning management phase often constitutes a problem at the beginning of the practicum since the students have to motivate themselves for this particular type of practicum and also to prepare their physical and psychosocial environment. Then, during the practicum, it is more the in-depth reflection and especially at the abstract conceptualisation level that brings up learning problems. The questions to be answered daily in the logbooks are derived from the expected behaviours in each phase, then becoming an aid for the individual learning process.

Clinical supervision, as defined historically by social workers, involves a formal process of on-the-job support by a professional who is not in a position of authority to the particular supervisee. This form of clinical supervision during professional practice is not well established in North America but seems to be gradually taking place within the United Kingdom, as described by Fowler (1996). The Dumas tool is considered as a strategy for lifelong learning as it promotes growth in any professional who uses it as a self-assessment tool of her day-to-day practice. In fact, I have used it during clinical supervision sessions of nurses working in a community health centre in Western Quebec. The behaviours depicted by the tool help the supervisees to get in touch with what is needed to achieve in-depth reflection of their day-to-day experiences and so to become autonomous. These practitioners perceived the presence of a mentor (supervisor) as beneficial, but also realised that it was unrealistic for everyone to expect such supervision on a regular basis. This is why learning how to use the Dumas tool was considered to be as important as learning the process informing it. The tool appears to provide a strategy for practitioners to become autonomous in their own reflection-on-action so that in the future they will be able to reflect-in-action, as suggested by Schön (1991).

Reflecting on personal experience helps one to find meaning from daily professional experience. It facilitates the professional growth of nurses by helping them to learn how to accept the joys, the excitement and the satisfaction whilst also gaining new understanding. Such learning can be tested in practice and hence consolidated within the practitioner's own frame of reference so as to enable her to use such knowledge in a variety of other settings as needed. By reflecting on what she does in her day-to-day practice, a nurse can advance from a technician to a professional, since not only can she perform with excellence but she can also give reasons for her practice.

Appendix to section 3.8
Excerpt from the Dumas Tool

Reflective observation phase

This is a phase during which the learner objectifies what emerges from the concrete experience, allowing the practitioner to make observations and reflections (descriptions, interpretations, evaluations, patterns) directly related to a particular experience and, sometimes, to other personal experiences of the experiences of others. In this component, the learner is still intimately involved in the immediate experience which may also be connected to previous experiences.

Behaviour to be evaluated in this component	Scale of performance	Anecdotes
	1 2 3 none	
14. Strives to describe her recent experience from the vantage point of an observer. *Indicator:* Strives to suspend her action in order to question it, withdraws sufficiently from the experience to be able to observe it objectively.		
15. Strives to explain the relationship between her experience and the resulting reflections. *Indicator:* Strives to report her experience faithfully; attempts to provide precise descriptions; strives to establish an accurate link between the experience and her observations.		
16. Identifies patterns or regularities in the current experience or through several experiences. *Indicators:* Recognises a pattern in this experience and previous personal experiences; 'I always thought that...'; 'I always did...'; reports similar or different patterns from others.		
17. Expresses a judgement on the experience and/or its effects in relation to the intention to act. *Indicators:* Judges elements of her entire experience; evaluates the emotional impact of the experience on her motivation and self-esteem; the issue is the intention to act, not to learn, which belongs to the learning management field.		

References

Benner, P. (1984) *From Novice to Expert*. Addison Wesley, Don Mills, Ontario.

Bennett, J. & Kingham, M. (1993) Learning diaries. In *Nurse Education: A Reflective Approach* (J. Reed & S. Procter, eds) Arnold, London.

Brookfield, S. (1987) *Understanding and Facilitating Adult Learning*. Jossey Bass, San Francisco.

Brookfield, S. (1987) *The Skillful Teacher* Jossey Bass, San Francisco.

Burnard, P. (1983) Through experience and from experience. *Nursing Mirror* 156 (9), 29-33.

Burnard, P. (1991) *Experiential Learning in Action*. Avebury, Brookfield.

Charbonneau, B. & Chevrier, J. (1990) L'apprentissage expérientiel, fondement théorique et cadre d' étude du savoir-apprendre expérientiel chez l'adulte. In *Les actes du 9e congrès annuel de l'Association Canadienne pour l'Étude de l'Education des Adultes* (B.S. Clough, ed.) Department of University Extension and Community Relations, University of Victoria.

Deane, D. & Campbell, J. (1985). *Developing Professional Effectiveness in Nursing*. Prentice Hall, Reston, VA.

Dumas, L. (1995) Élaboration et validation d'un instrument d'évaluation formative de la démarche de savoir-apprendre expérientiel de l'infirmière-étudiante en étage clinique. Doctoral thesis presented to the Université du Quebec à Montréal for the grade of PhD in Education, Interdisciplinary Program, June.

Dumas, L. (1997a) A tool to evaluate how to learn from experience in clinical settings. Oral and poster presentation at *8th Annual International Participative Conference on Nurse Education Tomorrow, Networking for Education in Health Care*, University of Durham (England).

Dumas, L. (1997b) Étage en soins infirmiers auprès des individuels, course SOI 5163 syllabus and notes for the students, Hull (Quebec, Canada): Université du Quebec à Hull.

Etienne, A. (1991) Du choix d'une approche pedagogique en fonction de la philosophie disciplinaire. *Revue de pedagogie de l'enseignement superieur* 10 (1), 5–15.

Fowler, J. (1996) The organization of clinical supervision within the nursing profession: a review of the literature. *Journal of Advanced Nursing* 23 471–8.

Kolb, D. A. (1984) *Experiential Learning. Experience as the Source of Learning and Development*. Prentice Hall, Englewood Cliffs.

Krikorian, D. A. & Paulanka, B. J. (1982) Self-awareness: the key to a successful nurse–patient relationship? *Journal of Psychiatric Nursing and Mental Health Services* 20 (6) 19–21.

Manley, M. J. (1997) Adult learning concepts important to precepting. In *The Role of the Preceptor: A Guide for Nurse Educators and Clinicians* (J.P. Flynn, ed.). Springer, New York.

Palmer, A.M., Burns, S. & Bulman, C. (1995) *Reflective Practice in Nursing*. Blackwell Science, Oxford.

Schön, D. A. (1991) *The Reflective Practitioner: How Professionals Think in Action*, 2nd edn. Jossey Bass, San Francisco.

3.9   EXPERIENCES OF SUPERVISION IN A PRE-REGISTRATION NURSING DEGREE COURSE

Sally Ballard

Having quite recently completed my preparation for registration as a nurse I am going to explore a particularly rewarding experience of supervision. This experience took place during my final year of training and almost at the end of my programme. It was at a time when I was especially sensitive about my performance as a nursing student – which is as a supervisee in the supervision process. I will use reflection to explore the experience. It was encouraged throughout my nurse training. Reflection can be described as a way of turning experience into learning. There are a number of frameworks on the process of reflection. Atkins & Murphy (1993) identified three key stages to the frameworks they analysed. Stage one in the process is awareness of uncomfortable feelings and thoughts. Stage two is critical analysis of the situation. This stage involves analysis of feelings and knowledge. The final stage is that of finding a new perspective on the experience. In this way learning has taken place. New knowledge has been integrated with existing knowledge. I will use this generic structure as I explore my experience of supervision.

Critical incident

I was in my fourth and final year of the adult nursing degree and this was my final placement ward. It was a 26-bedded ward for the rehabilitation of older people. Older adults who have been ill often need more time to recuperate before they return to their original level of independence. My objective for this final term was to begin to work at the level of a newly qualified staff nurse. I needed to take on the caseload of a member of staff (taking into account my ability and experience). I would then have to demonstrate the skill of managing this caseload throughout my shift, both in terms of the personal needs of individual patients, and in terms of planning and executing my work across the caseload.

On this particular shift my workload included admitting a lady to the ward. She was 87 and had recently suffered a stroke. This had left her with a reduced ability to speak and swallow. She was also left with a significant weakness in her right arm and leg. The lady's daughter and son-in-law were present when the patient arrived on the ward. I introduced myself to both the patient and the relatives. One of the first things I explained was that I was a student on the ward working under the supervision of a mentor. My badge clearly stated my student status, but I always felt it important to clarify this so that my position was clearly understood.

This elderly care ward had features that were useful to me. The relatively slow nature of admissions and discharges to the ward meant that they could be planned. My mentor and I had time to plan for this admission. We knew in advance the type of patient we would be receiving. My mentor and I made a point of discussing this forthcoming admission. We discussed the types of problem she was likely to have. We agreed the role I would play in the admission and the care I would undertake. I felt confident to admit the lady and complete the paperwork and, able to speak with both the patient and relatives about the aim of this admission. It was possible that this lady would need a naso-gastric tube. I had seen a naso-gastric tube passed on a number of occasions but I had not practised it myself. My mentor and I agreed that I could pass the tube with direct supervision from her. My mentor then left me unsupervised throughout the admission process. I spent considerable time with the family talking about the general health needs of the patient as well as the changes that had arisen from this admission. Whilst I was with them, my mentor agreed that she would oversee the other patients in my workload.

I had a fairly healthy level of anxiety about this admission! I was at a stage in my training at which I wanted to demonstrate to myself and to my mentor that I could act as an autonomous practitioner. I wanted to do everything for the patient and be able to answer every question that arose. This might have been an unrealistic goal to set myself, given my relative inexperience, but I wanted to feel confident that I could act alone. I felt that I wanted to manage the overall situation and therefore prove to myself that – yes – I was good enough to qualify as a nurse in a month's time! In this way the worries I had were exaggerated because I was putting pressure on myself. I felt that there was a clear distinction between the unqualified and qualified nurse, and I was trying to leap the gap between the two. My anxieties also arose out of the unknown nature of the admission. Every admission is unique because every patient and their circumstances are unique. Whilst I felt I had knowledge about strokes I was aware that my knowledge was limited. Any detailed questions the family might have about length of recovery I was not so confident to handle. Similarly I did not know how the family would present themselves to the ward. They would no doubt be anxious, but this anxiety might present itself as aggression towards me. I was anxious that I might find myself in an uncomfortable situation.

I am aware that much of my anxiety was related to the newness of the situation I would be confronting. The reflective process is all about learning from experience. But at this stage I felt that I had little experience from which I could learn! My mentor was well aware of my concerns. She could sense my nervousness at dealing with this situation on my own, yet understood that I wanted to act independently. The time we spent together planning for the admission was invaluable. We talked about how I would conduct the admission: what questions I would ask; what information I would give out. It was during this time that I could draw on my mentor's knowledge and experience to fill in the gaps of my knowledge. We talked about how she might handle a situation if the relatives were hostile or angry. Much of the time my mentor made me describe the stages of the admission. In this way she was helping me to articulate my thoughts. It then became apparent to me that I knew more than I thought I did! I just needed the confidence to put this knowledge into practice. I had admitted patients on other wards, so the process was not new to me. But I was still at a stage where I was not confident to adapt the skills I had from one situation to another.

For me, an overriding feature of this clinical supervision situation was the relationship between my mentor and myself. I needed, and we achieved, what I would describe as a good working relationship. I had confidence in my mentor, and respect for her nursing abilities. Similarly I agreed with many of the strategies she put forward for dealing with situations. Whilst I did not want to end up a clone of my mentor, our approaches had to coincide. If they were too dissimilar I would not feel able to adopt her suggestions. My confidence and respect for my mentor stemmed from working with her throughout the placement. I had observed her in a number of situations at the beginning of the placement. I was impressed by her knowledge and by her interpersonal skills. She had worked on the ward for 7 years and was now a primary nurse. She had a diploma in care of the older adult. I could see that she put her knowledge into practice, and she was willing to share it with me. She was a good role model to me. The time we spent talking was invaluable. We achieved open and honest communication during which I felt able to express my concerns and she felt able to give me feedback on my ideas and decisions. These talks gave me insights into the clinical work of nursing, but also gave me tremendous support in the emotional work involved. Cahill (1996) did a study of nurses' experiences of mentorship and found that a major feature that enhanced student learning was a supportive relationship between student and mentor. The students benefited more when they were supported by their mentor rather than controlled by them. I feel that these features were present in the relationship I had with my mentor. I felt supported by her. She showed respect for me by allowing me to express my ideas and opinions. She allowed me to negotiate the role I would play rather than dictating to me how I would work.

I can relate my experience to the idea of legitimate peripheral participation (Spouse 1998). In legitimate peripheral participation a new nurse works with an established nurse in acquiring nursing skills. In this way the experienced nurse 'sponsors' the new nurse. The experienced nurse introduces the new nurse to the community (in this case the ward) and helps to establish their credibility and identity. The new nurse works on peripheral activities at first, but then slowly acquires more skill and status. Legitimate peripheral participation is described as a joint enterprise. The new nurse and the experienced nurse work together to complete a case-load. I can relate much of this theory to my experience. My mentor and I were working as a team. My mentor's confidence on the ward meant that she was able to be flexible and allow me to take on as much work as I felt I could manage. In each shift I could renegotiate the extent of my role for the coming shift. She would accommodate this and take on the remaining work herself. I took part in legitimate activities on the ward. I did not feel that I was given minor tasks to do. Instead I was allowed to complete significant and legitimate pieces of work. In this way I was achieving competencies for myself, and completing work for the ward. I felt credible to the patient and relatives, and to the other members of staff.

Having taken the time to plan for the admission I then felt so much more confident to undertake it alone. I felt I had a solid foundation from which to work. I was still nervous, but my anxiety was reduced. I have to say that I found the experience rewarding as I felt that I was being given responsibility to act alone, whilst knowing that I had the support of my mentor behind me. That was probably the key feature for me about my supervision. I felt supported and valued. My mentor achieved this by treating me as a legitimate member of the team, and by allowing me to share her nursing work. Underpinning this was a strong relationship that my mentor and I had developed. We had open and honest communication. I was allowed to speak and express ideas. My mentor was willing to share her knowledge with me and give constructive feedback on my performance.

References

Atkins, S. & Murphy, K. (1993) Reflection : a review of the literature. *Journal of Advanced Nursing* **18** (8), 1188–92.

Cahill, H. (1996) A qualitative analysis of student nurses' experiences of mentorship. *Journal of Advanced Nursing* **24** (4), 791–9.

Spouse, J. (1998) Learning to nurse through legitimate peripheral participation. *Nurse Education Today* **18** (5), 345–51

3.10   REFLECTING ON PRACTICE IN SUPERVISION

Lisa Benrud-Larson

When asked to contribute to this book by writing about a critical incident I had experienced during supervision, I must admit that I was a bit hesitant at first. Throughout my education I had not had a great deal of exposure to the notion of critical incidents in teaching/learning. As such, my first task was to do a bit of background reading. According to Tripp (1993), the term 'critical incident' historically referred to some event or situation which marked a significant turning point or change in the life of a person or institution. Tripp (1993) goes on to say, however, that in teaching or learning situations, critical incidents typically are not unique and sensational occurrences but, instead, rather commonplace events which occur over the course of one's regular professional life. These common events become critical incidents only through one's reflection and analysis of the events and the subsequent meaning assigned to them. Such reflection often culminates in recognising the original event as characteristic of more underlying or general trends or motives (Tripp 1993). Armed with this definition, I began thinking about my experiences in supervision. My goal was to delineate a number of situations or events, which I considered to be critical incidents in the sense that they contributed to my training as a psychologist and resulted in an effective learning experience.

As a recent graduate of a PhD program in clinical psychology, I am no stranger to supervision. Actually, I might argue that the quality and effectiveness of my clinical training has depended to a large extent on the quality of supervision I have received throughout my various clinical experiences. As one might expect, in six years I have encountered many different supervisors and supervisory styles, some effective and some not so effective. As I think about it now, the supervisors I felt to be most effective were the ones who encouraged the use of reflection during and in between our supervisory sessions. In fact, I believe that reflection is a crucial aspect of supervision if one wants to learn the most one can from one's clinical training.

Looking back over the past six years of my training, I can think of several critical incidents which contributed to my professional growth as a clinician. I believe, however, that I benefited most from the clinical supervision I received during my internship year: the final year of my predoctoral training. I completed my internship at a large teaching hospital where I received regular supervision from several licensed psychologists. This usually consisted of weekly one-on-one meetings with the psychologist who was supervising the rotation I was completing at the time. The supervisory meeting would typically last for one hour during which we would discuss my current caseload. I learned a great deal from each of my internship supervisors and could probably write about any number of learning experiences I had with each of them. The critical incident I have chosen to write about revolves around the supervision I was receiving on a particularly challenging individual psychotherapy case.

The individual I was working with was a single, middle-aged, Caucasian woman (Ms R.) who had been referred for psychotherapy by her physician. She had recently been hospitalised due to progressive physical decline secondary to a muscular disease. The referring physician was concerned about Ms R's mood and had prescribed an antidepressant for her. He also thought that psychotherapy might be beneficial in helping her adjust to her increasing disability. Before meeting Ms R. I reviewed her chart on which the physician had noted that she was having difficulty adjusting to her physical deterioration and progressive loss of independence. Upon meeting Ms R. I did an initial assessment and determined that she was experiencing several depressive symptoms, including depressed mood, anhedonia, disturbed sleep and appetite, decreased energy and concentration, and feelings of worthlessness. As had been noted in her chart, she was having difficulty adjusting to her increasing disability and subsequent loss of independence. Ms R. had lived alone most of her adult life and she hated the idea of having to become dependent on someone at this point in her life.

Ms R. and I began meeting regularly for psychotherapy. Initially, she reported an improvement in mood and she appeared to be making some progress in adjusting to her current physical status. Further into treatment, however, Ms R. experienced more physical setbacks and a subsequent increase in the severity of her depressive symptoms. She began experiencing regular suicidal ideation accompanied by a vague plan of how she might hurt herself. At this point I talked with Ms R. about a contract for safety in which she would agree to contact me or the local emergency department immediately should she feel she was in danger of harming herself and before she acted on those thoughts. Unfortunately, Ms R. only vaguely agreed to the contract, stating that she would try to follow through with the terms of the contract should she find herself in that situation. At that point I made the judgement that this was sufficient at that time, coupled with an agreement that we would meet again in three days instead of waiting a week between sessions as was our typical pattern.

It was at this point in the therapy case that supervision became critical to me. Although I had been meeting regularly with my supervisor throughout the period I was seeing Ms R., at this point I began consulting her even more frequently. I specifically recall telephoning my supervisor immediately after the session during which Ms R. and I had discussed her safety and the need for a safety contract. My supervisor was out of her office at the time of my call, so I left a message for her to call me back as soon as possible as I would like to discuss an issue with her regarding one of my clients. I am sure there was more than a small amount of concern in my voice! My supervisor called me back promptly, as was her tendency, and I proceeded to explain my concerns regarding what had just happened in my session with Ms R. As one can imagine, I had several concerns. I was concerned not only about my client's safety, but also about my responsibility to do everything in my power to assure her safety. Had I done enough? During my education I had read and heard a great deal about what one should do in a situation like this. However, as a beginning clinician, I still had not encountered many such cases. As such, I was feeling very unsure of myself.

My supervisor and I talked a great deal about this situation, both during my initial telephone call to her and during later supervisory sessions. Looking back now, I would say that these discussions were critical in teaching me more about who I was as a clinician. My supervisor always made use of reflection during our supervisory sessions. During our first discussion regarding Ms R's suicidal thoughts, I went over the details of the session and commented that I was unsure whether I took the appropriate steps to protect the safety of Ms R. My supervisor did not immediately reassure me that I had acted appropriately (as I had hoped she might do), but instead had me reflect on what I had done and why. Upon reviewing the choices I had made with Ms R. as well as options I did not pursue (e.g. hospitalisation), I felt more confident that I had acted responsibly and appropriately in my role as Ms R.'s therapist.

Only after going through what I had done and why, did my supervisor state that she supported my actions and likely would have acted similarly if put in the same situation. I realise now that telling me this after I had come to that conclusion myself was a much more effective use of supervision than if she had told me immediately that I had acted appropriately regarding Ms R.'s situation. By having me reflect on the reasons for my actions, my supervisor helped me to discover that I did have the knowledge and training to handle the situation and, even more importantly, that I was able to put that knowledge and training to use when necessary. Had my supervisor immediately reassured me, I likely would not have gone back through my actions and reflected on why my choices were or were not appropriate. Instead, I may have breathed a sigh of relief that I had 'lucked out' and acted appropriately with Ms R. on that occasion. I probably would have continued to doubt that I really knew what I was doing as a therapist and, therefore, likely would have felt no more confident that I could handle a similar situation in the future.

Despite this boost in confidence and our conclusion that I had taken the necessary steps toward protecting the safety of my client, I was still feeling uneasy about the situation. Thus, during my next meeting with my supervisor, she had me think back over my session with Ms R. and report all the feelings I was experiencing during and immediately after the session. The goal was to try to determine why I might be feeling so distressed if, as we had discussed, I had taken reasonable and appropriate steps to protect my client's safety given the circumstances of the case. We first discussed that it was normal to feel uneasy in a difficult situation such as working with a potentially suicidal client. In fact, it would be worrisome if I was not concerned about the welfare of my client. As we continued to discuss the situation, however, I discovered more about what was at the root of my uneasiness.

In discussing specific feelings I was experiencing regarding this situation, I kept going back to the same ones: fear/anxiety, doubt, and helplessness. I was afraid that my client's safety was at risk and still anxious about whether or not I had not done enough to ensure to a reasonable degree that she would not hurt herself. In line with this, I was anxious about my level of responsibility should she hurt herself (would her family hold me responsible and consequently pursue a malpractice case against me?). The fear and anxiety were tied directly to considerable feelings of doubt regarding my competency as a therapist. Although I knew differently, I felt that if I was a competent therapist I should have been able to cure my client or fix her problems. Her depression should not have been worsening; it should have been improving. I must have been doing something wrong. A more competent therapist would have been able to help her. One particular thought that had entered my mind on more than a few previous occasions kept running through my head: I really did not know what I was doing. Perhaps this profession was not for me.

All of these feelings were accompanied by a general sense of helplessness. I felt I had no control over the situation. Again, I had the sense that if I really knew what I was doing, I would have a better handle on things; the situation would not feel so out of control to me. I would know what to do to ensure my client's safety. If only there was a book to tell me exactly what to do!

In talking more about this with my supervisor, I concluded that this sense of helplessness I was experiencing was related to my general uncomfortableness with ambiguity. I have always been a person who likes structure. For example, in college I preferred the courses that were mapped out clearly from the beginning. I knew exactly what I had to do for the course and what was expected of me, and was able to prepare accordingly. In contrast, I never liked those classes that tended to be more free flowing: the ones where the professor would often go off on a tangent during a lecture and never quite return to the scheduled topic. This need for structure, of course, was quite naturally incorporated into my graduate training. For example, as a therapist-in-training I sought for control in therapy sessions through the use of structured approaches. I am quite sure that my uneasiness with ambiguity is, in part, what attracted me to a more structured school of therapy.

My supervisor helped me relate this need for structure back to my anxiety regarding my competence as a clinician. I suppose my belief was that if I always adhered to a type of therapeutic approach which was described clearly in several texts with accompanying examples of specific techniques and strategies, then I would easily be able to learn how to be a good therapist. Similarly, if I always structured the therapy session, there would not be much room for ambiguity. I would always be prepared. I would not need to think on my feet, so to speak.

As I stated above, these supervisory sessions were critical in terms of helping me learn more about who I was as a therapist. In particular, they helped me recognise areas on which I needed to concentrate during supervision (e.g. increasing my confidence and spontaneity during the therapy session). One way my supervisor and I agreed to work on these areas was through the use of videotaping (a tool which greatly facilitates reflection). With the use of videotapes, we were able to observe together my actions during therapy sessions and to stop and discuss specific sections as appropriate. For example, I might identify an area where I remembered feeling as though I did not know what to say or do. My supervisor would then have me reflect on what was going through my mind at that point. Next, we might discuss why my course of action was or was not appropriate in that situation, and brainstorm alternative approaches I could have taken at that point in the session. In addition, my supervisor regularly reinforced actions that she viewed as evidence of my competence as a trainee, whether that was good use of empathy during a session, utilisation of an effective intervention, or timeliness in paperwork. Looking back now I believe she did a good job of utilising any negative or positive emotions I was feeling regarding my work/performance as a clinician. For example, she was able to help me learn that the many negative emotions I was experiencing (e.g. fear, anxiety) were in part acting as barriers to my learning in the sense that they were resulting in a desire to give up rather than to use the emotions constructively. At the same time, my supervisor was able to bring out any positive emotions I might be experiencing and use them as an impetus for me to continue in what I saw as a challenging situation (Boud *et al.* 1985).

The issues that I have discussed (e.g. lack of confidence in my abilities as a therapist) had arisen to some extent during my sessions with other supervisors; however, we never seemed to work on them as much as I did with this particular supervisor. I believe there are several reasons for this, some of which I have already discussed (e.g. effective use of reflection). First, my supervisor was very approachable and available to me. Whether I had a scheduled meeting or caught her on the run in the hallway, she always made me feel as though I had her full attention. In contrast, some other supervisors I had worked with tended to give the impression that I was using too much of their time. For example, they might regularly cancel meetings, be late, cut meetings short, or fail to return telephone calls in a timely manner. Second, this supervisor was very supportive and empathic. In providing such a supportive learning environment, she made supervision a very non-threatening and effective experience rather than one that I faced with dread. Third, this supervisor achieved a good balance in the amount of direction she provided. She allowed a great deal of independence, but at the same time offered direction when needed. In my situation, she was careful not to offer too much direction as she likely knew that, if she did, I would simply employ what she suggested versus thinking things through on my own.

This supervisor definitely helped me learn how to use supervision effectively. Prior to working with her, I tended to dread supervision. I did not want to reflect on my actions and feelings for fear that my supervisor (and I) would discover what a terrible job I was doing. She was able to remove the threat I associated with supervision by handling everything in a very sensitive manner. As a result, I was able to reframe my view of supervision as a helpful learning experience and begin to use it to my advantage. Candy and colleagues argue that the aim of reflective learning is to develop learners who are capable of monitoring themselves (Candy *et al.* 1985). I believe this is exactly what the supervisor I have been focusing on in this paper did in my situation. First, she helped me recognise the importance of reflection in learning, and second, she helped me develop the ability to monitor my actions and feelings in a variety of situations; a skill I will undoubtedly utilise for many years to come.

References

Boud, D., Keogh, R. & Walker, D., eds (1985) Promoting reflection in learning: a model. In *Reflection: Turning Experience into Learning*. (D. Boud, R. Keogh & D. Walker, eds), pp. 18–40. Kogan Page, London.

Candy,. P., Harri-Augstein, S. & Thomas, L. (1985) Reflection and the self-organized learner: a model of learning conversations. In *Reflection: Turning Experience into Learning* (D. Boud, R. Keogh & D. Walker, eds), pp. 100–16. Kogan Page, London.

Tripp, D. (1993) *Critical Incidents in Teaching: Developing Professional Judgement*. Routledge, London.

Chapter 4

Case Studies of Supervision during Organisational Change

4.1 THE IMPACT ON SUPERVISION OF MOVING FROM HOSPITAL TO COMMUNITY

Ann V. L. Davies, Paul Simic and Janet Gregson

This case study arises from reflections on regular supervision sessions between two occupational therapists, Ann and Janet, who worked as supervisor and supervisee respectively. Over a three and a half year period we engaged in approximately 50 sessions of structured discussion. Our local trust had obtained some central government funding to create a new multi-disciplinary community mental health team. Premises were rapidly found and staff moved at a similarly rapid pace with little regard for the dynamics of the project. Social workers and community practice nurses had already moved from other locations to this base. Janet, who had worked as a mental health occupational therapist for 10 years in the local hospital, was recruited to the team. Following the project initiation there had been little time to plan how the team would work together. Instead the team had a naïve faith in the magical effects of common roof space on promoting joint working and learning.

Context of the service

Currently there is, in the caring services and the public sector generally, a lowering of morale. The new National Health Service structure has brought threats to professional practice from general management and the consumerist culture. It is no longer sufficient to hope that treatment or therapy is effective: it has to be proved and be seen to be cost-effective into the bargain. Occupational therapy in mental health is facing the same demands, for example, as the nursing profession. These have been identified in the Sainsbury report, *Pulling Together* (Sainsbury Centre 1998) as a need not just to move physically from institutional settings to the community but to change ways of thinking and working practices. This requires moving from institutional and hierarchical approaches to more flexible, innovative and empowering ways of thinking and working. It is in the light of these changes and insecurities that we write. As with other professions there has been and continues to be a fundamental debate about the roles and responsibilities of occupational therapists and the critical defining aspects of practice that distinguish them, particularly when seen from the health care purchaser/commissioner point of view, from the other providers.

Occupational therapy is a predominantly female profession and has just less than 10 000 representatives registered with the Council for Professions Supplementary to Medicine. The last 20 years have seen radical changes in the way services are delivered and the role of the patient or 'user' therein. These changes have done much to challenge traditional roles and thinking in relation to professional stability. As an 'emerging' profession (Blom-Cooper 1989) it is possible that occupational therapy has had more challenges to its identity than others which are more established. The World Federation of Occupational Therapists defined occupational therapy as the treatment of physical and psychiatric conditions through specific activities to help people to reach their maximum level of function and independence in all aspects of daily life (Blom-Cooper 1989). This is achieved through both purposeful activity and occupation (Golledge 1998a,b). Hagedorn (1995) describes four central elements that comprise the core of occupational therapy. These are person (as in patient), therapist, occupation and the environment within which this triad operates. Hagedorn contends that the placing of the first three in an interactive environment is a feature of occupational therapy. There is also nothing esoteric about the occupational therapy focus. Most of us tend to take for granted everyday tasks such as talking to a stranger or visiting the toilet. But these tasks in the context of disability can be anything but routine and anything but simple. The occupational therapist is able to analyse a problem and, using her knowledge and skill, can construct some means of overcoming a problem by relating it to the needs of the patient. Often this is in conjunction with the patient. The target group for the service was people with more serious and intractable conditions. This served to justify the relatively low caseload numbers that were labour intensive. Some clients received two to three lengthy visits every week for very basic skills training. Very quickly it was found that the occupational therapy input to the mental health project was subject to a greater demand than anticipated. The amount of time available to spend with clients remained a bone of contention. Pressure from general management to fulfil contact numbers put pressure on practitioners to spend less time providing quicker but less effective interventions. What appeared to be teething problems became entrenched and fixed ways of working and relating, which hindered any effective development. As with all developing teams in which structures are not fully in place and the team is operational without sufficient preparation and planning, operational problems were brought back and fed 'upwards' for resolution. For example, no physical boundaries were agreed for the team. Social Services operated with different boundaries to health from those observed by the health-employed occupational therapist, and even from those of the community psychiatric nurse (CPN). There were problems in taking inter-agency referrals. Sheer persistence from social work colleagues might have resulted in out-of-area referrals being taken just to improve referral rates (and in a sense to improve relationships) but the supervision process allowed careful consideration of the pros and cons of such practices.

The nature of supervision

There were no formal outcome measures defined for the OT service in the community but the monitoring of informal peer review was recognised as critical. As in other caring professions, professional supervision of occupational therapists is a core part of professional development and quality assurance. Perceptions of supervision, its function, quality and mode no doubt vary greatly amongst practitioners. Supervision can reinforce the quality issue and give permission for the adoption of an appropriate clinical role such as challenging some of the worst aspects of an attitude dominated by throughput considerations rather than care. In the context of this case study, the emerging pattern of supervision was of meetings being held on an *ad hoc* basis in response to urgent requests. They were informal and lacked an agenda. Frequently they were concerned with some clinical work such as approaches to treatment or with management issues of caseload numbers, problem cases or case descriptions which led on to discussion about roles and responsibilities. Much of the supervision was based around referral rates; sources of referral and a need to advertise the service to generate appropriate referrals. Latterly within the supervision sessions the emphasis on referrals and contacts diminished as more important operational problems took precedence and as the project became more established. The content of the supervision began to incorporate a mix of information downward in terms of policy, legislation and new developments. Weir (1991) suggests that occupational therapists need to keep up to date with these issues in order not to be left behind. This process emerged as a natural progression to the supervision. Content of the supervision activities can then be summarised as having three main elements:

(1) Practical – actual monitoring aspects of practice, caseload numbers and giving permission for cases not to be taken on.
(2) Professional – ensuring the maintenance of a clear role, again 'permission' to take on certain tasks or take on certain responsibilities.
(3) Political – steering a professional role ensuring future practitioners and practice gain from the experience of this supervision. This has much to do with operational management of teams and the interface between team managers/co-ordinators and clinical/professional managers.

The changing model of supervision

Both of us had worked within the same hospital setting for many years. We had an established line management relationship that was based on mutual respect and friendship. It therefore seemed quite natural for Janet to go to Ann for professional support following her transfer into the community setting. The professional isolation and the unstructured and unfamiliar approach to practice necessitated opportunities to 'touch base'. The first point for discussion in reflections on the style and pitch of supervision between supervisor and supervisee was whether there was in fact a different model being employed after Janet moved into the community setting. We agreed that Janet could contact Ann whenever she needed supervision support. The sessions were not structured or pre-planned and did not include any form of formal arrangement such as a contract, action plans or reflective journals. This lack of structure made it much easier for Janet to seek professional support and to tease out issues concerning her role. The management experience of Ann meant that she could share her professional knowledge and provide some guidance on role boundaries as well as reinforce Janet's own approaches to managing her experiences. As these issues became less important Janet began to use the supervision differently. Both of us felt strongly that there were distinct and unambiguous changes, which were identified as being both shared and idiosyncratic to each of us. This change was articulated in terms of a perceived shift from a hierarchical model to a horizontal, more facilitative model:

'I felt that we moved from discussions solely around my cases to a shared focus on my own role and development.' *(Janet)*

This change was reflected in the nature of the discussions and their focus. Whereas in the early stages Ann had been able to provide information and guidance, the discussions became concerned with collaborative problem solving and opportunities to rehearse strategies or plan arguments before meetings. This approach to professional development has greater meaning for Janet as it has helped her to develop a range of important personal and professional skills. If the sessions had been formalised, through contracts and action plans, it is unlikely that the relationship could have developed to one of 'critical companionship' (Titchen 1998). One regret has been that neither of us used a reflective journal or diary to record our experiences.

Craik (1998) describes research from the United States, which as in our case reflects the profession's reliance on a medical model and the fact that occupational therapy remained hospital-based when mental health services moved into the community. The flattening of the hierarchical model is also due in part to changes in working location and team structure. Community mental health teams rely on close team working and it is probably true to say that most have not achieved the 'real team' model described as the ideal (perhaps too ideal) by Ovretveit (1992). Even the best laid plans cannot or do not account for inter-professional and inter-agency conflicts, interpersonal problems, administrative difficulties and the gamut of operational problems encountered and engendered by these in day-to-day working. Supervision outside the team in a clinical/professional context is important in resolving some of these difficulties, particularly for less experienced clinicians. Craik *et al.* (1998) in a survey of 200 OTs working in mental health found that of the 137 respondents the largest group were Senior I staff aged between 20 and 30 years. Nine per cent had worked in mental health less than 5 years and 68% for less than 10 years. Team membership or time in current post tended to be significantly less than actual time in practice. Of the respondents 82% had been in their current post less than 5 years and 23% less than 1 year. This implies that unless the occupational therapist had previous experience of working in teams their post tended to be a relatively new community experience for them. This perhaps reflected our own experiences of the transition from hospital to community as a new venture, although Janet was an experienced occupational therapist in mental health. The research highlighted the diversity of duties carried out by occupational therapists in teams. This may reflect a deliberate adoption of a generic mode of working in a team that Janet was trying to resist, but may also reflect the inexperience of a clinician in developing an occupational therapist's specific role. The presence of a team manager or co-ordinator (both different roles) means that clear pathways of responsibility and accountability need to be defined and agreed in order to make supervision effective and to be of the greatest benefit to the practitioner.

The determinants in community settings for this changing model

The determinants of the change model are implicit in the move from a hospital to a community setting. This represents a shift of focus for occupational therapy from a medical to a social care model. This was felt to be the core determining feature of the change of ethos in supervision to a more empowering and supportive model. The move has been from the traditional occupational therapy department, often uni-professional. The occupational therapist is often single-handed, relying on team support and 'team-playing', working to a social model that demands autonomy and innovation. Working within this model but still obtaining direction and identity from one's own profession is fraught with difficulty yet opens up the potential for occupational therapy practice in the future. We would argue that this shift from a hierarchical to a more democratic model necessarily involves a similar shift in the model of professional supervision. Accountability and quality issues remain just as central but the means of getting there are different. The supervisor has to be more facilitative and more supportive than a traditional authority figure and 'fount of all knowledge'. This shifts the balance, or perhaps more accurately redistributes the weight of the respective contributions of case and service management requirements in the supervision process. A greater emphasis is placed on individual professional development. This includes the development of professional and personal skills that may involve assertive but collaborative task skills and what might be termed public relations skills.

Unlike a hospital setting, the community service is too amorphous a concept to take any reinforcing identity from the local community mental health trust. Perhaps it is too frail. This means that solidarity with a professional identity is more critical in the increasingly public milieu of interdisciplinary team working in the community. All the issues interweave, the more covert as well as the overt aspects of professional supervision. This includes the warp of creating an identity with the health provision setting (hospital or community), as well as the weft of professional identity (medical or mental health occupational therapist), to reconstruct the fabric of supervision into a new model.

Lessons

We wish to draw out some lessons for supervision practice and for occupational therapy. Supervision in this context acts as a marker, a point of reference for occupational therapists working in the community and in multidisciplinary settings. The discourse around the limits to occupational therapy – what an occupational therapist should and shouldn't be doing in that setting – forces both supervisor and supervisee to reflect on the core competencies of their profession and its ethical and philosophical stance. There is no reason in principle why this should not (and may well) happen in more institutionalised settings. But where the structure of the care model is more prescriptive (where power is held in fewer hands) and where traditional ways of working create the inertia characterised by attitudes depicted as 'this is how things are done', innovative and proactive thinking are stifled. The shift into a more flexible and social model nevertheless requires experienced practitioners who feel secure in their role and with the limits of their skills. It may be worth noting that an essential back-up for any occupational therapist is the professional code of ethics and conduct, which also states the limits of the professional role. The Sainsbury Centre for Mental Health Research (Onyett *et al.* 1995) found that occupational therapists have high team identification but low professional identification. The supervision process should aim to guard against this conflict, although it may engender some anxiety for the team member in terms of asserting a professional identity. It may be that core members of the team such as the community psychiatric nurses and the social workers are already well established and have preconceived ideas of the role of the occupational therapist which may contribute to any anxiety.

The supervision process can also relate to the vexed question of team versus professional management, where lines of accountability and authority (for want of better expressions) may be unclear and agreement has not been reached in any planning phase. Mention has already been made of the need for clarity in this issue, particularly where supervision may be provided within the team. Is there a role for professional supervision? We would argue that there is if the occupational therapist role is to survive in future.

What have we learned personally? The supervisor would have found valuable the use of a reflective diary or at the least some record of the supervision process. This would have helped to clarify the management decisions that needed to be made about the post (of supervisor) and would have been useful in supporting the post-holder through what has been at times a traumatic and far from easy process. Looking back over three years for the purpose of this narrative the supervisor is surprised and impressed by the change in the supervisee's skills and experience. The transfer of occupational therapy core skills to a new clinical setting has left me far behind as a hospital-based practitioner. The supervisor's own learning and experience have been acquired as a manager making difficult decisions about the configuration of the service and negotiating on behalf of this colleague to facilitate her role as a practitioner as she carved a niche for herself and for the profession.

References

Blom-Cooper, L. (1989) *Report of a Commission of Inquiry, Occupational Therapy: An Emerging Profession in Health Care*. Duckworth, London.

Craik, C. (1998) Occupational therapy in mental health: a review of the literature. *British Journal of Occupational Therapy* **61** (5) 186–92.

Craik, C., Chacksfield, J. D. & Richards, G. (1998) A survey of occupational therapy practitioners in mental health. *British Journal of Occupational Therapy* **61** (5), 227–34.

Golledge, J. (1998a) Distinguishing between occupation, purposeful activity and activity, Part 1: Review and explanation. *British Journal of Occupational Therapy* **61** (3), 100–5.

Golledge, J. (1998b) Distinguishing between occupation, purposeful activity and activity, Part 2: Why is the distinction important? *British Journal of Occupational Therapy* **61** (4), 157–60.

Hagedorn, R. (1995) *Occupational therapy: Perspectives and Processes*. Churchill Livingstone, London.

Morgan, S. (1996) *Helping Relationships in Mental Health*. Chapman & Hall, London.

Onyett, S., Pillinger, T. & Muijen, M. (1995) *Making Community Mental Health Teams Work*. Sainsbury Centre for Mental Health, London.

Ovretveit, J. (1992) Concepts of case management. *British Journal of Occupational Therapy* **55** (6), 225–8.

Sainsbury Centre for Mental Health (1998) *Pulling Together*. Sainsbury Centre for Mental Health, London.

Titchen, A. (1998) A conceptual framework for facilitating learning in clinical practice. Occasional Paper No. 2, Royal College of Nursing Institute, Radcliffe Infirmary, Oxford.

Weir, W. (1991) Emerging from behind closed doors. *Australian Occupational Therapy Journal* **38** (4), 185–92.

4.2 SETTING UP SUPERVISION IN MENTAL HEALTH AND LEARNING DISABILITY SERVICES

Lesley Rudd and Philip Wolsey

This second case study addresses the strategy formulation and strategy implementation issues which were involved in an 18-month project to design, build, implement and evaluate a Trust-wide system of clinical supervision for nurses and health care assistants. The Trust was a large mental health and learning disabilities Trust in Surrey (England). The group of staff who were to be involved was wide-ranging, including, as it did, graduate professionals working at the highest clinical grade level ('G' grade), along with people working at 'A' grade for whom English was not their first language and who were working as health care assistants. Many staff in the Trust had received no professional development for many years. In two of the pilot sites there was a strong union culture and a great suspicion that this was a management tool with a sub-agenda for weeding out poorly performing staff. This was an early indication of the pejorative connotation that the word 'supervision' has for many people and one reason why we adopted the words *supervisor* and *practitioner*. An important consideration was the introduction in 1995 of the policy regarding Post Registration Education and Practice (PREP) by the United Kingdom Central Council for Nurses, Midwives and Health Visitors (UKCC, the statutory professional regulatory body for nurses). This required registered nurses to give evidence of undertaking the equivalent of five study days every three years as a condition for their continuing registration to practise.

During the 18-month life of the project the Trust was going through an enormously turbulent period. This political dimension impacted severely on the project during months 10–18 and in effect stonewalled the introduction of supervision in several clinical areas. This political dimension has to be both recognised and understood because unless a project of this size has constant champions at all levels and in all places, it will not succeed. Such champions have to keep pushing and chivvying throughout. When jobs are on the line and in the gift of non-(clinical) professionals, even the most committed of souls will turn from their convictions. Many of these people are not convinced that supervision is worth the time, money and effort. There is little empirical evidence to show the link between supervision and improved outcomes for patients.

However, there is national and international evidence of improved morale and reduced levels of sickness as a result of clinical supervision. But much more research needs to be done. Nurses' commitment and conviction need to be backed up with substantive evidence that is difficult to come by in busy overstretched nursing services. Our audit of what had been achieved indicated that there was a substantial improvement in patient outcomes.

In this case study we give some of the reasoning behind what has been developed as well as some detail of how to do it. From the beginning we were determined to be able to show the positive effects of supervision on patient care as well as to develop a system that would be (and is) valued by nurses and their representatives. There are many interested parties who use and who pay for nursing services, so we aimed through the audit mechanism to show that effective supervision can add value and security for patients. The case study discusses the following crucial implementation questions:

- What is a suitable model for supervision when the concept is still relatively immature in nursing?
- How do you get the money and other resources for such a project?
- How do you deal with the change management issues?
- How do you evaluate the impact on outcomes?

Background to the project

Surrey Heartlands had a very chequered history. It was a single Trust consisting of two units, one concerned with caring for people with learning disabilities and the other for people with mental health problems. The Trust had emerged only in 1994 and each of the separate units had made previous attempts at achieving Trust status both alone and with other suggested partners. The income base was around £42 million in 1995. The culture in each unit had been very different but both had suffered from chronic underfunding. The staffing levels were poor and a blame culture prevailed. At the time of merger there was a climate of suspicion between the two sets of staff; some lack of confidence in the managers; some alienation of the staff-side representatives and a rapid turnover of clinical directors. Having said this, there was a general desire to move forward and to share knowledge. This was particularly true of the professional nurses within each unit. Surrey Heartlands had over 1200 staff on the nursing grades. It had a long history of limited development opportunities for staff who were consequently poorly motivated to change. There was also a major hospital closure programme underway. A Nursing Policy Group had been formed in early 1995. It was a thriving group of representatives from all parts of the nursing service, a representative from Human Resources (personnel), and one from the union. This group was authorised by the Executive Directors of the Trust to undertake work and to implement as well as to make decisions about nursing practice throughout the Trust. To meet the requirements of the executive the Group wished to provide assurances for all our stakeholders (clients, commissioners, educators, advocates and carers) that we could provide safe, up-to-date and outcomes-based care.

In wishing to introduce supervision the Nursing Policy Group was responding to national and professional initiatives coming from the NHS Management Executive and the UKCC (National Health Service Management Executive 1995; United Kingdom Central Council 1996). It was also determined to improve the quality of the clinical environment and thus the quality of the service provided to clients/patients and their carers. In so doing it recognised the current disparity and fragmented nature of the Trust's residential and community services as well as the lack of support that staff received whilst providing care under increasingly stressful working conditions. It was anticipated that a more co-ordinated and focused approach could be developed to improve clinical practice and the skills and competencies of the staff, whilst supporting professional practices of autonomy, accountability, critical thinking and reflective practice. The members of the Nursing Policy Group realised that there was no ideal model of supervision and decided to develop a local model that fitted their needs and those of their patients. It wanted to ensure that staff received both support and feedback in their practice, which challenged some current thinking in a safe environment. Initially we had not thought through how the project would develop but had agreed the concept and that we should aim for Trust-wide introduction. If this was achieved by staff who were more committed, with better attendance levels and who felt supported by their peers and managers, so much the better. We were also convinced that we had to be accountable for the results of the project and the financing that we had to secure. The subsequent concentration on money provided additional encouragement to design an audit tool of the outcome of the project.

Resourcing the project

Financial resources

It immediately became apparent that the project was going to be a long piece of work, concerned as much about changing the value base of the organisation as about introducing a new system. This meant that the project would be expensive in terms of use of both human and financial resources as well as of the energy of the project working party. The facilitation and training of staff and supervisors would be expensive and the audit would also take time and resources. The theme of cost was a long-running issue throughout the project. At the time of this project we were hampered by our inability to convince the sceptics and the money-men that supervision would have any payback. Whilst this is a criticism easily levelled at non-clinical people it is also a criticism of professional colleagues. Although the climate is now changing with the introduction of clinical governance, we still have to find a substantive way of demonstrating how cost effective supervision can be (see Ellis 1992; Holloway & Neufeldt 1995; Butterworth *et al.* 1997). When we eventually devised the model of supervision that we wanted, we costed our initial introduction of supervision at £300 000 in the first year. This was to be found from existing resources. We were able to argue that through effective supervision we could save money by reducing levels of sickness, currently at 7%, and incidents of malpractice, which might result in lengthy and thus costly litigation. In these days of very limited resources it is not acceptable to rely on blind faith in a system of supervision, and we needed to produce evidence of its effectiveness. People have many legitimate questions about how we spend taxpayers' money and whether we spend it in the most cost-effective manner. Our interpretation of cost effective was that of improved outcomes for patients.

The Nursing Policy Group started the project by exploring possible sources of funds, and several things conspired to help us. An important factor was the recent introduction of a more localised and accountable system of nurse education in the National Health Service. This was moving the previous system of funding nurse education from regional offices to a local education unit. It was nearly the end of the financial year and our unit responsible for contracting education services had spare funds. It was keen to support the project and so the Trust secured enough money to engage a management consultant with experience of developing supervision in health care settings to facilitate the project. The selection was made against several criteria:

- The project needed someone who knew and understood the clinical culture and the working environment
- We were seeking someone who was as totally committed, perhaps even evangelical, towards supervision as ourselves
- We were also seeking someone who could introduce rigour, who had a knowledge of research and who had some considerable empathy for our situation

The project working party

At a meeting that all the senior nurses in the Trust attended, the outline of the project was explained. After much open debate we identified and agreed on four different parts of the service as volunteer pilot sites to trial the introduction of supervision. From this meeting we set up a project working party, which was chaired by a senior nurse (practice development) and composed of enthusiasts selected from across the Trust representing each pilot site. These practitioners represented staff from a long-stay ward for older people with mental illness; a community mental health team (CMHT) for people with general psychiatric illness; a home for severely physically and mentally disabled people and a home for people with mild autism. Other members of the working group were senior development nurses, senior quality specialists and nurses from the wards and the community. It was agreed that this project working party should be kept to 10 nurses. A management consultancy agency (OPDC) was commissioned to facilitate the project working party. Its consultant, Phil Wolsey, joined at the outset with a notional commitment of 40 days over a year. We realised that this would be a process of huge change for all of us and that it might involve some difficult times. We did not want the process to be undermined by having any other external members of the working party. By good fortune we discovered that we had a good mix of team player types (Belbin 1981) and this was invaluable in providing robust, rigorous work which was also delivered on time. So important was this good team mix that the following year, when we moved to an Implementation Steering Group, we felt we could not continue until we had the one team member who asked all the challenging questions. The working party was required to report through its chairperson to the Professional Nursing Group. Although the executive nurse would not be a member of the group, the project continued to be led and driven at executive level. This helped overcome barriers on several occasions due to the leverage that executive sponsorship affords, and was key to progress.

The working party devised the project plan and set to work agreeing a definition of supervision. It also agreed a number of operational issues such as time scales, communication strategy, target dates, training and support plan. The group obtained some baseline data and devised questionnaires for stakeholders. Ideas could then be further debated as required and ratified for action.

The approved objectives of the project working party were to:

(1) Implement a structured pilot programme of supervision in four clinical areas. This would include:

- setting standards for supervision and methods for evaluating its effectiveness
- undertaking and delivering training in supervision and audit
- establishing trainers and cascading the training
- undertaking a series of activity analyses

(2) Set up a system which would address the metrics of quality of service, cost and speed of delivery of health care complete with methods of measurement and data collected
(3) Support and restore practitioners when constantly working with stress and distress
(4) Identify and involve the key stakeholders crucial to the success of the project

Developing the model of supervision of practice

The nature of the project required us to ensure that we had a firm grounding on which to establish our approach. Over the first 12 months we reviewed the literature to ensure that the approach related to the best accepted practice. This literature review helped us to set the fundamental principles, to set standards of practice within supervision and to develop and implement the model of supervision that we wanted for the pilot sites. We also had to write the documents for introducing supervision and auditing its effect. These documents were regularly reviewed and updated in the light of feedback we received. Wide communication of our activities was an important part of the process and included holding open sessions for staff as well as writing reports and articles on the project. The total commitment and results from the working party were a clear example of excellent co-operative working. More than anyone the members moved the whole culture of the organisation. We also undertook some research within the Trust and found some one-to-one supervision already under-way within the community services. This was patchy, disorganised and unfocused, and offered (mostly) support but little challenge.

Developing a model of supervision

The working party set out to devise a definition of supervision and a model that would suit all the staff working in these four clinical areas of work.

A fundamental activity was to agree on a definition for supervision and what we were trying to achieve. We recognised that both formal and informal approaches to supervision are essential for effective clinical practice and that setting up formal systems of supervision in no way supersedes or replaces the informal systems. We developed a definition which required an approach that was planned in advance, had a formal contract which specified the timelines and the work to be done and which was written in such a way that made its provisions specific, measurable, attainable, relevant and trackable (SMART). We aimed to introduce a system that over the medium to long term, would promote practitioners who would develop skills of analysis, reflection and autonomy, and who would be able to use the literature to inform their thinking and their practice. This was in preference to people who relied upon others to provide solutions. These aims required a more structured approach that could only be achieved through a formal system of supervision. This would encourage practitioners to develop an analytical approach to their practice and to develop their self-respect and confidence.

We believe that many people fear supervision because in their minds it is associated with criticism of their practice far more than it is associated with validation of it. Inevitably it is the case that if anyone looks at our practice they will find flaws in it and as a result it is difficult not to take criticisms personally. Whilst we know intellectually that people need praise, validation etc., what we tend to notice and give attention to is that which jars us. This results in more notice being given to the extremes of good and bad practice rather than to small examples of routine good practice. Research on appraisal systems suggests that people are disabled by as few as three critical comments of their work (Latham & Wexley 1994). Writing about her research into staff attrition in hospital settings, Isabel Menzies Lyth (1988) indicated the unhappiness created by such approaches:

'...the traditional relationship between staff and students is such that students are singled out by staff solely for reprimand or criticism. Good work is taken for granted and little praise given. Students complain that no-one notices when they work well, when they stay late on duty or when they do some extra task for a patient's comfort.'

The same may be true for all grades of practitioners, and clearly there is a nettle to be grasped here. How were we to reassure practitioners that supervision will be a supportive exercise whilst at the same time, where necessary, reserving the right to challenge fearlessly and unsentimentally, anything which is unsound, unsafe, ethically dubious or even illegal? It is essential that poor practice should be highlighted if we are to discharge our responsibilities to patients/clients, their carers and to the taxpayer. We believe that the purpose of supervision is to deliver high quality healthcare, which is a wider issue than episodes of care. We identified four key elements that informed the concept of clinical supervision: support, standard setting, skills development and personal development (see Table 4.1).

Table 4.1   Key elements of supervision of practice model

---

(1) *Support*

In the course of their work practitioners accumulate stress and distress as a consequence of coming into contact with people who are in psychic or physical pain. If this is not dealt with, it can lead to levels of stress which create problems for the practitioner, leaving her or him 'shut down' and uncreative. Long-term problems can be extreme, culminating in serious errors, burnout and even early death (Cherniss 1980). Well managed supervision sessions will leave practitioners feeling lighter than when they came in. We refer to this as a process that restores the practitioner (Proctor & Inskip 1989).

(2) *Standards Setting*

Supervision is a form of quality assurance and therefore a part of clinical audit. It is designed to deliver high quality health care. The aim is not merely to help practitioners achieve high quality standards of practice but also to maintain those standards once achieved.

(3) *Skills Development*

Supervision can offer opportunities to rehearse critical situations, to try out different ways of dealing with phenomena and to receive feedback that will enable practitioners to build incrementally their skills and ideas about how to deal with various circumstances. Within supervision sessions practitioners could practise a range of scenarios which are causing difficulties, e.g. interviewing a patient; confronting a colleague; rehearsing a tricky performance review; making a presentation to a fund holder about service provision; or giving a talk to students or staff in the local Faculty of Health. These examples are intended to illustrate our view that the role of a practitioner in delivering high quality health care is more than direct patient contact.

(4) *Personal Development*

This is one of the most sensitive areas in which a supervisor may provide support and challenge. It is important to be clear about boundaries. Here supervisors help practitioners to understand the impact of thinking on personal behaviour and the impact of behaviour on patients, clients and colleagues. It is a sensitive area because it is often perceived to involve our personalities, sensibilities, defences and motivation (conscious and unconscious) and may feel just a bit too psychological for our comfort. It is not intended to provide therapy.

Defining the principles

The working party members planned that supervision of practice would be set up to provide professional support and development for all practitioners (i.e. all qualified and unqualified nursing and care staff) working in any of the services provided by the Trust. This would be achieved by enabling practitioners to discuss their practice with a trained supervisor in either prearranged or 'live' supervision sessions. Supervision of practice would be in addition to statutory requirements for student mentorship and preceptorship offered to new staff. We agreed that supervision would take place in an internal healthcare system and be paid for by the taxpayer, i.e. that it would take place within working hours rather than within the practitioners' off-duty time. We also identified that it would be flexible enough to integrate into a multidisciplinary system and would emphasise research-based practice and clinical outcomes. Supervisors would be expected to use their knowledge and experience to assist practitioners to think about and to develop their skills, knowledge and values to provide consistently high quality care to patients and clients in a process which included support, challenge, skill development, maintenance or improvement of standards and personal development. This approach to supervision of practice would aid registered nurses to meet the requirements of the UKCC for continued registration and would contribute to clinical risk management through ongoing review of practice. These principles would make *supervision of practice* part of the professional culture of all nursing staff employed by the Trust.

The model of supervision of practice would ensure that every practitioner would have 10 hours' supervision per year (pro rata) irrespective of holidays. This could be provided in a variety of ways, i.e. it could be live, live-delayed, peer group or one-to-one supervision. An essential aspect of the supervision was the use of supervisory contracts, which had to be negotiated and agreed by both practitioner and supervisor. Such contracts would include ground rules describing the manner in which the supervisory relationship would be conducted, and would include statements about confidentiality. Issues of importance could only be discussed outside the supervisory session with the agreement of both parties. This was designed to promote a climate of confidence and trust that we believed was essential to encourage an attitude that criticism was welcome. We recognised that the confidentiality issue is a very contentious issue that few organisations may feel able to sign up to. The working party also argued that anything that affects issues outside practice must be discussed in supervision, and agreement reached as to how it could be taken further. Records of supervision would be kept and would remain in the ownership of the practitioner. Such records would only be used as a reminder of what was discussed and of the actions agreed.

This work all became enshrined in a clinical risk management policy for the Trust, and the supervision entitlement for the different grades of staff is listed in Table 4.2.

Table 4.2   Supervision entitlement of staff by grade (level of commitment made by the Trust

---

Nurse grade A/B/C/D will:
- receive 10 hours per year (pro rata) in direct supervision
- be involved in 22.5 hours' (3 days pro rata) training on supervision per year

Nurse grade E/F/G will:
- receive supervision and be supervisor
- receive 10 hours per year (pro rata) in direct supervision
- undertake 40 hours per year as a supervisor (to four practitioners each)
- be involved in 45 hours' (6 days pro rata) training on supervision per year

Nurse grade H will:
- receive supervision (possibly peer) and be supervisor
- receive 10 hours per year (pro rata) in direct supervision
- be involved in 100 hours per year as supervisor (a maximum of 10 practitioners and supervise the supervisors in group sessions)
- be involved in 90 hours' (12 days) training on supervision per year

Nurse grade I/SNP will:
- receive 6 hours per year (pro rata) in direct supervision
- be involved in 40 hours' per year as supervisor
- be involved in 45 hours' (6 days) training on supervision per year

---

Training supervision trainers

It is not cost effective to give 1200 practitioners training in supervision delivered by external trainers. The project working party decided to use a cascade or domino approach to training supervisors. Having identified a dozen or so credible practitioners, our management consultant trained them to work as supervision trainers. These people would not only be able to deliver the formal training inputs but would also act as local experts who were on tap to answer questions and to give ongoing guidance after training was completed. We discovered in the pilot trials that this local expert resource was crucial in keeping the implementation of supervision on track. Those practitioners who received more supervision than they would be giving (e.g. health care assistants) received a half-day input so that they would be familiar with the model and would share a set of common assumptions. The training of trainers took a total of 15 days and involved supervising their practice of preparing others during their training sessions. This was intended to give them support in their presentational and group work skills whilst being credible. Other important skills that they needed to feel confident about were the ability to answer tough questions about supervision and to process the group whilst ensuring they covered the curriculum. We also arranged that both the trainers and the supervisors could receive academic credit for their work from one of the local universities.

Auditing supervision of practice

Since introduction of the internal market in health care, many groups of people have joined the list of stakeholders who are concerned with effective practice and thus with supervision of practice. These stakeholders are all looking for assurances that supervision improves health care outcomes, raises standards and gives practitioners the support that is so often lacking in these busy days. Like all customers they will measure these improvements in terms of quality, costs, levels of service and reduced cycle times for key activities. In devising an audit tool we were keen to ensure that it reflected the measures that the various stakeholders would deem important.

The audit process

We devised audit standards based on data gathered from stakeholders. The detailed audit process itself drew heavily on approaches used in the quality management system ISO 9001 (British Standards Institute 1994). To achieve this we consulted as widely as possible using a questionnaire that we devised and by interviewing a selection of people from all the groups of stakeholders. We identified these as being patients or clients, carers and advocates, practitioners, supervisors, education providers, service commissioners, staff representatives (union representatives), and senior managers.

From this audit activity we found a consensus among all those approached. Their concerns were that the service should be of a high standard and that it should be monitored rigorously and without sentiment. They were also concerned that practitioners should be safe, supported and challenged or stretched, but not subjected to stress. This required a fair process which improved the welfare of the staff whilst developing their talent and potential to achieve career development. Such development should reflect high standards of professional research-based care, congruent with the strategic direction of the trust and with professional matters. In particular the senior management wanted staff who could think imaginatively as well as strategically about health care as a business and beyond a narrow professional view. The development of knowledgeable practitioners and high standards of care would improve the quality of the service. Practitioners would also reflect critically on their practice whilst constantly modifying that practice in the light of current research to the benefit of clients and patients. In this way they would provide good mentorship support for students, thus increasing the benefits of having more learners placed in the clinical areas.

From our audit findings we were able to demonstrate that our practitioners were developing the ability to use research to inform their practice and as a result our facility to assess clinical risk was becoming more refined. We were keen to gather compelling stories on the lived experience of supervision and to show the links between supervision and practice. To this effect we trawled the contracts of supervision to identify clauses in the agreement, which were clearly aimed at clinical interventions. We then audited the record of supervision to see how the clause was progressed in the supervision session(s), and went on to the clients' care plans to see the link between them and the supervision session. Finally, the auditors asked the client and family what they thought of the intervention. Whilst this process could not establish cause and effect, it provided compelling anecdotal evidence of the link between the work taking place in supervision and the final outcome for the client.

Conclusions

This project showed us how very difficult it can be to implement supervision throughout an organisation without a considerable number of very committed vocal champions. It can be a huge change for any service. The current political emphasis on clinical governance will have an impact. But most managers, even those with a clinical background, are beset with pressures from all quarters to use resources differently and as a result clinical supervision has not been a priority. We found that initially practitioners can be extremely wary of professional supervision. This changes when they have training in supervision and have personal experience of good supervision. At Surrey Heartlands, where supervision was introduced and embraced with enthusiasm, it still continues. The early audits of care plans showed improved outcomes for patients and greater job satisfaction and morale amongst staff. The greatest validation was that, during the pilot phase and when time was pressing, staff were still engaged in supervision outside their allocated work time. Whilst this was far from ideal and not to be recommended, it did provide us with evidence that commitment to and desire for supervision by practitioners were very strong.

The contract with OPDC was completed and both of the authors subsequently left Surrey Heartlands. A new management structure now exists as a result of a further merger with another Trust. It is reputed to be committed to implementing supervision Trust-wide for the whole nursing service. The exercise of implementing supervision of practice, although difficult, very time consuming and occasionally frustrating beyond belief has left us even more firmly convinced that supervision done well and supportively is key to improving services and to ensuring a well motivated and competent nursing service. We owe a great debt to the working party members and to the trainers who worked so hard to make supervision of practice a reality. We also acknowledge with gratitude the practitioners who over many months were prepared to participate in the pilot trials. Without their commitment, enthusiasm and persistence we would not have been able to develop such a robust and successful system for our service.

References

Belbin, M. (1981) *Management Teams: Why They Succeed or Fail.* Heinemann, London.

British Standards Institute (1994) BSEN ISO 9001: *Quality Systems. Model for Quality Assurance in Design, Development, Production, Installation and Servicing.* British Standards Institute, London.

Butterworth, T., Carson, J., White, E., Jeacock, J., Clements, A. & Bishop, V. (1997) *It's Good to Talk.* School of Nursing, Midwifery and Health Visiting, University of Manchester.

Cherniss, C. (1980) *Burnout in Health Service Organisations.* Praeger, New York.

Ellis, M. V. (1992) Research in clinical supervision: revitalising a scientific agenda. *Counsellor Education and Supervision* 30, 238–51.

Holloway, E. & Neufeldt, S. (1995) Supervision: its contributions to treatment efficacy. *Journal of Consultant Clinical Psychologist* 63 (2), 207–13.

Latham, G.P. & Wexley, K. N. (1994) *Increasing Productivity through Performance Appraisal.* Addison-Wesley, Wokingham.

Menzies Lyth, I. (1988) *Containing Anxiety in Institutions: Selected Essays.* Free Association Books, London.

National Health Service Management Executive (1995) *Priorities and Planning Guidance for the NHS: 1996/97.* Department of Health, London.

Proctor, B. & Inskip, F. (1989) *A Working Alliance.* Video tape and manual from: 4 Ducks Walk, East Twickenham, Middlesex.

United Kingdom Central Council for Nursing, Midwifery and Health Visiting (1995) *Standards for Post Registration Education and Practice (PREP).* UKCC, London.

United Kingdom Central Council for Nursing, Midwifery and Health Visiting (1996) *Position Statement for Clinical Supervision for Nurses, Midwives and Health Visitors.* UKCC, London.

Chapter 5

Supervision of Clinical Practice: The Nature of Professional Development

Jenny Spouse

Throughout our professional lives we have opportunities to learn. This continuous expansion of knowledge provides a sometimes overwhelming body of information on which to draw. Working in a community of practice enables everyone to contribute and to draw upon each other's expertise, irrespective of how long they have practised. As a result we are all learners whilst at the same time being in a position to offer supervision at some level to our colleagues. Such an approach requires an ethos of mutual value and openness to sharing. Some experienced practitioners have a wealth of craft knowledge which may sometimes be difficult to describe in formal or academic language but which can be shared through their skilled practice or through their narratives of practice with clients. This chapter sets out to explore how such craft knowledge (Brown & McIntyre 1993) can be communicated to enhance the professional development of others through a close supervisory relationship. The critical incidents described in Chapter 3 show us the fundamental importance of a good interpersonal alliance. A more subtle note to these narratives is the value of having regular opportunities to observe experienced practitioners, to be coached by them and to have opportunities to practise independently. This practice needed to be followed by pre-planned debriefing times for reflection and discussion of observations of practice and personal activities. Such opportunities for discussion worked best with a trusted and knowledgeable practitioner who was able to encourage the 'learner' to share her or his thinking about the experiences. Lisa Benrud-Larson in Chapter 3.10 described her encounters with a supervisor willing to engage in such a dialogue and suggests the rarity of such experiences. In exploring these critical incidents or case studies of supervision, I shall be drawing upon available evidence from recent research on nurses' professional learning and the influence of supervision. Much of this is based on a study investigating the acquisition of professional knowledge by nursing students (Spouse 1998a). A second source of evidence comes from work by Angie Titchen exploring nurses' development of work-based, experiential knowledge (Titchen 1998). Earlier discussions of a student–mentor relationship (Spouse 1996) have relevance to every supervisory relationship and they been developed further using a range of material taken from educational and social theories.

In discussing students' experiences of learning to become nurses it is suggested that their experiences bear many similarities to those of any practitioner wishing to develop their professional expertise, whether they are working in a new clinical setting or in one that is familiar. This is particularly true for newly qualified practitioners moving into their first job or moving into an unfamiliar practice setting. Even experienced practitioners changing their clinical workplace setting or practice speciality are likely to share the same difficulties at first. Initial unfamiliarity with local or specialist terminology and daily activities and facing old problems presented in different guises requires translation of professional knowledge to the new context as well as development of new forms of professional craft knowledge. Many practitioners carry a wealth of craft knowledge borne from considerable experience, which they are able to adapt to a new area of practice and to their new setting. Nevertheless in the early stages of transition to a new setting they will still require help to make adjustments and to settle into their new environment. In everyday practice the complexities and expectations of everyday health care practice compound the demands of personal growth and change with the rapid developments caused by technology and growth in understandings of health and illness. Such developments are challenging and require constant vigilance and professional updating. Their complexity is further compounded by the special nature of professional endeavours incurred by working with people of all ages, social backgrounds and experiences of health and illness. Learning to recognise and to respond effectively to such complex ranges of health care needs collaborative learning activities and opportunities to discuss and develop ways of responding effectively. This can only be achieved when practitioners work in an environment that fosters critical enquiry and support. This chapter seeks to address several questions that preoccupy most people offering supervision. In particular the questions are concerned with the nature of the relationship between supervisor and supervisee; the characteristics of effective supervision; the way in which professional development can be promoted and, not least, how such processes may be implemented.

Studies of women in learning situations demonstrate that environments which foster images of self-worth encourage students to develop a strong identity as successful learners (Hallsdórsdóttir 1989; Conrad & Phillips 1995; Ingleton 1995). Pre-registration nursing students in my study demonstrated that environments of this nature freed their energies to concentrate on learning rather than to worry about managing the strong emotions of loss and isolation. Their good experiences relate to learning in traditional communities of practice which exist in many non-indus-trialised settings and where both children and young adults are appren-ticed to expert craft workers and where the relationship between learner and teacher is close and supportive (Rogoff 1990, 1995). Such relation-ships are more in tune with a warm and nurturing learning climate where emotional deterrents to learning such as fear and shame do not even begin to enter the relationship. In these communities participants are handled sensitively and affirmation is considered paramount. Lave (1991) identi-fies a three-point model in effective apprenticeship of *membership, socialisation* and *learning* where *participation is peripheral and legitimate.* Building upon her own studies and those of Rogoff, she argues that cognition is only possible through involvement in communities of practice, and uses a range of examples concerned with adult learning to demon-strate the effectiveness of a structured and respected place within the community (Lave 1991). Her work has relevance for nursing and other health care learners as it enables newcomers to learn from old-timers in a manner which can be responsive to students' needs (Spouse 1998c). It is a more sophisticated process than that labelled as role modelling and, rather than distant supervision, it requires the student and teacher to work closely together. The first step in developing such sponsorship is through giving the newcomer a legitimate role within the community which gives access to learning opportunities. As the student comes to feel secure within the relationship and in the setting, the burden of responsibility shifts from an intense relationship between learner and sponsor/mentor and is shared among all the staff who are perceived to be approachable. With good befriending, learners are more likely to recognise and to use coaching opportunities and to develop their professional understanding. Such attunement, the respected educationalist Jerome Bruner argues, enables learning to become spontaneous and memorable (Bruner 1986). It seems clear that the ideal learner–mentor relationship contrasts radically with the more common experience, based on remoteness and competitiveness and identified as being alienating and destructive.

The transition from a system of education where learners were apprentices and part of the workforce to the current status of being pre-dominantly a supernumerary learner, emphasises the importance of a mentor. Students' presence in clinical areas on a short-term, individually negotiated basis leaves them more dependent upon their mentors for support. It is also possible that encounters with caring for sick and needy patients are so unfamiliar and frightening that the only way to survive is to have the support, and in some instances the protection, of an experienced practitioner. Its absence in earlier programmes of professional development may well account for the large attrition rate experienced by nursing, and also raises questions about the quality of care that can be delivered. Many experienced practitioners benefit from opportunities to review their professional practice during a supportive relationship as in the critical incidents described by Charlotte Chesson (Chapter 3.4) and Louise Dumas (Chapter 3.8). Some like Dave Roberts are able to draw upon past experiences to guide them in their reflections-in-practice. But this may not always be sufficient, as the practitioner in Barbara Lovelady's critical incident discovered, and this is when more formal support and education are needed through the sponsorship of an experienced supervisor.

Entry to the practice setting

Research shows that, despite introductory discussions and opportunities to meet the clinical manager for their placement, learners report feelings of confusion and bewilderment at their unfamiliar experiences and a sense of alienation that is related to the extent to which they feel part of a clinical team. Such feelings are natural when people are exposed to unfamiliar cultures, values, language, modes of dress and a different social structure. This painful process often requires a new approach to viewing self and to viewing personal relationships with other practitioners working in the setting. Newcomers need to learn how to behave in a manner that characterises them as members of their adopted community (the unfamiliar clinical environment). Students undergoing educational programmes that require frequent changes of placement are more likely to feel alienated owing to the short time they spend in any one place. Inevitably such frequent changes of placement mean they are allotted a different supervisor (clinical instructor, preceptor or mentor) in each new clinical setting and this disrupts any opportunity to develop meaningful relationships. With the current organisation of many professional programmes in higher education settings, learners are also faced with large student peer groups that undergo frequent changes, causing them to feel even more isolated. Certainly for the majority of their programme, all the participants in the research believed they needed to earn their place within each clinical team so as to legitimise the amount of time being used to support them. In most instances they felt they should undertake activities that were of use to the staff if they were to be exposed to learning experiences. Students believed this was a necessary strategy to repay staff for their efforts of teaching and tolerating them. Such feelings seem to be commonplace in any setting where newcomers feel a debt to the existing inhabitants. A similar feeling has been described by Wax (1952) working in unfamiliar settings whilst engaged in ethnographic research and where she was relying upon the good will of the local people for the success of her project. She describes this activity of undertaking beneficial activities as essential and named it reciprocity (Wax 1952, p. 36). Another researcher, Glazer, suggests that this process of reciprocating kindness and information is important as a means for gaining the trust of informants (Glazer 1982, p. 50). Students and any other newcomer to a clinical setting are reliant upon the same sort of good will from their colleagues or their supervisors who have the power to give or to withhold information. The critical incident below (narrative 5.1) provides a good example of how many staff feel when working in unfamiliar and hostile environments. In this situation it was written by a very experienced and educated practitioner working as an agency nurse whilst studying on a full-time postgraduate course:

> '[I] managed to support myself continuing to nurse at weekends. I really loathed it as [the] ward closed to yet *another* superb management re-organisation and ended up on orthopaedics. Too heavy and staff who worked there for 25 years plus seemed to find it quite unbelievable that anyone would not automatically know what to do in that field but also refused to impart any knowledge! They were extremely efficient but it seemed a very old fashioned notion or notions – both to stay in one hospital and indeed ward for so long and also to hug expertise to the detriment of care. The new grads totally loathed it most of the time. They were on a 3-month rotation for [their] first year and found it very difficult on that particular ward to find out what was expected of them and to develop skills, except in a hit and miss way.' (Maggie, 10 October 1997, Narrative 5.1)

As Maggie's narrative demonstrates, her experiences of being made to feel unwelcome, isolated and disempowered were shared by other visiting practitioners to this hostile ward environment. Evidence suggests this is not an unfamiliar experience for students who are often denied access to mentor support, resulting in similar feelings of loss and isolation (White *et al.* 1996; May *et al.* 1997; Spouse 1998a). An example of such difficulty is described by one learner in my research study (she has been called Marie). She was allocated for a period of eight days spread over four weeks to a childrens' ward. This was in the early part of her programme and she had arranged for me to observe her practice on the fifth day in the ward. During the observation period Marie's mentor involved her in washing a child's hair. It was the first time that Marie had been given care alongside her mentor or had been engaged in any structured learning activity with her. Until that day Marie had been left to get on by herself with her mentor trusting she would seek help if necessary. Following the period of observation the three of us discussed the observed activities and how Marie's mentor saw her role. I have called Marie's mentor Lilly, and this was her response:

'I find it very difficult. To me, my role is to show people what's on the ward, what's on offer, and talk about their experiences, discuss what their aim is and facilitate the other resources that we've got. And show them the other people on the ward, get the resources, teaching resources as well as books, and experience. We work very much as a team here. I don't know, I find being a mentor quite difficult, I suppose especially as I'm unclear about what it really is about. It depends very much on the person. The best thing is to do, if they're just happy enough to go and do things on their own.' (Lilly [Marie's mentor], interview 6b, Narrative 5.2)

Marie's mentor had not realised the significance of her relationship with a learner or how much help was needed to adjust to a new clinical area and to find a role. Lilly doesn't seem to have an image of herself working alongside the learner, sharing her nursing work, her decisions and her knowledge. Instead she seems to have seen herself as a signpost, directing learners to other people or resources. Marie's experience was compounded by her perception of the attitudes of many of the ward staff as she describes later when discussing her three different placements over the term:

'It was just so, like, "You're invading our [space] . . ." I just felt so out of place. "You shouldn't be here, what were you doing there?" Normally I find it really easy to talk to people and I just found it so hard, so awkward. I think if I'd have had a different response from the beginning, or maybe if my mentor had said "Well, I've spoken to so and so", or if I'd felt part of the team, maybe I would have been more ready to go along and say "Oh I'm here as a learner, I need to know X, Y or Z. Then I think . . . I just felt so totally alienated from the whole thing that . . . it didn't really make me want to work. I just felt, "Well, if you can't be bothered I can't be bothered".' (Marie, interview 7, Narrative 5.3)

Despite her assertions, Marie was clearly very upset about the way in which she had been treated. Like Maggie earlier, Marie felt her learning was being blocked and as a result she was unable to function effectively within the environment. Maggie's knowledge of the nursing organisation and her previous experiences as a ward manager gave her much more self-confidence and consequently she was in a stronger position to address the problem. Narratives from other practitioners and in the literature indicate how commonplace such experiences are and how much they detract from learning and professional development. In such situations the old-timers (the resident practitioners) are resisting acceptance of the newcomers (new students, new staff, agency/bank staff, etc.), and the sense of alienation which results characterises the concept of *Gemeinschaft* used in interpretive sociology.

Membership of a community

The interpretive approach to socialisation has a substantial history and provides valuable insights into understanding personal experience. The Chicago school of sociologists significantly influences our understanding of adult and professional socialisation – in particular the influence of Mead and his belief that, through seeing the self as an object, humans come to measure their ideal image and their actual performance against that of others (Mead 1934). Another important contribution to current understanding of adult socialisation has been the work of Brim & Wheeler (1966). These authors argue that role acquisition is the most important aspect of adult socialisation, and correlate it with personality change, as a profound and perhaps the most painful of adjustments made in life (Brim & Wheeler 1966). This process of socialisation requires learning how to make personal action come close to what is accepted as the norm for that community. Learning how to do this is believed to be achieved through social interaction and internalisation or absorbing the normal ways of acting pre-consciously. This is termed role-modelling by such writers as the psychologist Bandura (1977) and by Wiseman (1994) when calling upon Bandura's work to describe her observations of nursing. Learners' narratives in recent research indicate that they are concerned about the quality of practice they observe when working with other practitioners and recognise unsafe practice at an early stage of their course. This research indicates that students are more selective about who they choose to learn from than has been suggested by Bandura or Wiseman (May *et al* 1997; Spouse 1998a).

How people cope when beginning to work in unfamiliar settings has been extensively researched by a number of sociologists. Van Maanen (1976) drew upon theory from sociology, psychology and social psychology to support his investigations of socialisation. He uses concepts concerned with group membership and individual endeavour to explain differences in behaviour and expectations. The concept of group membership seems particularly useful in professional settings as it is concerned with a human desire to work towards becoming an integrated member of society, working on its behalf and thus learning to become one of the group. In achieving this state, new group members cease to feel exposed and vulnerable and enjoy the protection and support of their colleagues. One research participant in my study described her experiences of being a novice learner on a busy ward as behaving like a 'puppy dog' running behind her mentor. This illustrates her loss of identity and her dependence on her mentor in order to exist effectively (i.e. to learn and to be able to participate as she saw others participate) in the setting. Similarly she talked of 'nudging her way in with her elbows out' when she went to work in another clinical setting where staff left her on her own rather as Lilly did to Marie or as Maggie encountered on the orthopaedic ward. By contrast the concept of personal endeavour is associated with individual rather than team success and distinction. This allows them to operate independently of a community or a close network of friends and family (van Maanen 1977). The principles of personal endeavour are perhaps more apparent when people have the tools to pursue their own private aims, such as experienced practitioners operating independently or entering a new working environment where they have more control over their destiny and possibly the destiny of others. People who are dependent upon the support and co-operation of others in order to function, such as students and newly qualified clinicians, cannot survive in an environment where these principles operate. They require the closer communal support offered by peers in their settings. Without this support, being exposed to and adjusting to unfamiliar ways of behaving, a newcomer takes longer to settle in. Part of this process of socialisation includes being recognisable as a member of the group and conforming to existing patterns of behaviour, speech and dress if a newcomer is to become accepted. They must learn to dress like their new peers (e.g. wearing the same uniform as an occupational therapist or as a nurse or as a university student). They must learn the language, the jargon and terms that are only used by insiders of that setting – hence the need to become familiar with medical terminology or with the acronyms used by practitioners. Having someone who is willing to act as a 'key informant' or guide, someone who recognises the newcomer's dilemma and who is willing to explain unfamiliar terminology is an important means to settling in.

Adjusting to new settings may include learning how people relate to each other and this may be quite different from previous customary practice. Maggie's experiences of working as a relief nurse brought her into contact with unfamiliar working practices that conflicted with her own beliefs and values. Her encounters may have presented ethical and professional dilemmas that had to be resolved. On a less professionally disturbing level, the differences may be concerned with simple practices such as those encountered when visiting foreign cultures and where such behaviours as shaking hands or giving a kiss on each cheek on meeting are normal practice. In some clinical settings strict hierarchies exist whereas in others it is acceptable to call everyone by their first name. Newcomers need to be aware of such differences if they are to avoid making mistakes. They have to learn to accept such differences as part of getting used to the cultural expectations of their new setting. By learning all these new behaviours they become an invisible and accepted member of the team, no longer sticking out like a sore thumb. During their educational programme students are particularly exposed to a wide range of cultural settings due to frequent changes of clinical placement. Sometimes exposure to different attitudes and values can require radical changes in behaviour that communicate particular values. This following extract from a learning contract illustrates the point. It was written by a nursing student given the name of Helen, following her first nursing placement in her programme.

'I have had much experience with the elderly. However, my attitude has noticeably changed since my first few weeks working on the ward. One tendency was to treat all patients the same, and especially those with similar illnesses. However, having worked on the wards I have realised that each person should be treated as an individual as for example some elderly people have more self-respect than others. A simple example I found was that the majority of patients are called by their Christian names. It seems the accepted format. I met a new patient a few days ago and she introduced herself as Mrs Graham, as opposed to Anna, her Christian name. It made me realise that it is quite important to ask the patient what they like to be called when they first come to the hospital and not just assume that they like being called by their Christian name. Another patient may find it very formal and impersonal to be called Mrs, and this can be just as distressing for the patient. We must be aware of empowering the patient.' (Helen: Learning Contract: 270, term 1, year 2, Narrative 5.4)

This example may seem so simple and almost banal and yet for this student and for many other practitioners it heralded a significantly new approach to care giving: an approach that was taken for granted by the old-timers in the clinical setting and yet if she had chosen to ignore it, Helen would have been immediately distinguished as an outsider.

Sponsorship within a new culture

When newcomers or students feel accepted by their supervisor, they also come to feel more confident with meeting other members of the clinical team. This influences their ability to gain help for themselves and their patients. In placements where learners are able to work with supportive and insightful practitioners whilst delivering care to mentally or physically ill patients they gain a sense of self-worth, confidence and enthusiasm as the following narrative from a student whom I've called Gilles describes:

'I suppose this was the one thing, that it felt as though it was a partnership and I was involved in whatever, and how I felt confident enough to talk and people have listened to what I have to say. Before they've perhaps not listened to what you've had to say. Before, perhaps I didn't particularly know what was going on. Even in the ward rounds when people come, I'd chip in if I didn't agree with what was being said. People would respect what you said and take it on board. You felt you were being listened to, be it just as a student or a nurse, it was interesting.' (Gilles interview 10, Narrative 5.5)

Brim (in Brim & Wheeler 1966) argues that the most important influencing factors in the socialisation process are: frequent contact with members of the culture; their importance and their ability to create dissonance or well being in the newcomer. This supports the case for some form of supervision as being essential to newcomers to any (clinical) setting. Brim's assertions and the absence of effective supervision from many students' mentors explain their somewhat ambiguous situation in practice settings. Students in the studies identified earlier were neither integrated members of a nursing community nor members of the community of university students. This was due to the demands of their programme. Consequently they were left in limbo on their own. Essential to students' survival and success in their clinical placements was support from experienced practitioners who were knowledgeable and respected within the culture of their own practice setting and who could mentor students individually.

As the narratives of students in this research indicate, successful socialisation and thus integration with other members of the community depend upon the actions or responses of others for success. This is congruent with findings from a study of industrial workers by Nicholson (1987). He demonstrates that when newcomers are given peer and mentorship support, and are given clear instructions for their work and control over their work, they are more likely to stay than someone lacking such support and guidance when facing unfamiliar situations. Both the negative examples provided by Maggie and Marie and the good experience described by Gilles in Narrative 5.5 provide examples supporting Nicholson's findings. His research in UK industries demonstrates that change and adjustment are a cumulative process influenced by the extent to which workers are encouraged to implement their learning (Nicholson 1987). This reflects the expressed concerns of learners who often became frustrated by what seemed obstructions to their progress, and it could explain the loss of confidence and development of uncertainty in career choice leading some students or some staff to resign.

Supervisors in professional development

The fragmented nature of many professional programmes which are designed to prepare learners to recognise and to deal with increasingly complex practice makes effective support in clinical settings even more important. With the introduction of reflective practice or enquiry-based learning it is believed that learners will have access to practitioners who are able to discuss their practice. Such access makes effective supervision even more essential if practice is to be made meaningful and if students are going to learn how to relate propositional or formal classroom knowledge to their practical experiences (see Spouse 1998b).

Trusting your mentor

As Nicola so clearly states (p. 138), it is essential for learners to develop sufficient trust with their supervisors so that any limitations and learning needs can be identified and attended to. This can only be achieved when students feel confident with the guidance and support from someone they can trust. They also need to feel the person is sufficiently approachable to let them explore their feelings. Both Sally Ballard and Lisa Benrud-Larson (Chapters 3. 9 and 3.10 respectively) identified that their mentor should be someone who is sufficiently approachable to be asked questions. It is clear that some clearly defined form of effective supervision is essential to professional development and progress, irrespective of the status of the practitioner. The research data, and indeed the critical incidents presented in Chapter 3, demonstrate that the quality of a supervisory relationship is the most significant influence on professional development. As with most forms of supervision this relationship encompasses many dimensions.

Mentor's understanding of their role

Other practitioners with whom learners come into contact also influence their development to both a greater and a lesser extent but such encounters are facilitated by students' relationship with their mentors. It is possible that, like Marie's mentor (Lilly) earlier, and mentors such as Lorna and Charlotte in Chapter 3, many mentors and supervisors have not conceptualised their (new) role and this can result in practices that result in both student and mentor feeling isolated and unsupported.

Practice experience

A third factor influencing professional development is the nature of practice activities in which mentors are willing to engage their learners. This affects the extent to which learners are able to access professional or craft knowledge. Some mentors find it difficult to identify suitable activities for students during their placement or for a new member of staff who is unfamiliar with the setting or clinical practice. Often students are either left on their own or given tasks that are below or far beyond their capability. By contrast, in successful situations students are encouraged to develop skills within their development range and then permitted to practise them with effective distant supervision. Such opportunities provide inspiration and confidence. They also motivate learners to explore and develop associated theoretical knowledge about their case load with exciting results.

Characteristics of effective supervision

When investigating the relationship between learners and their mentors, four specific characteristics were identified from the research data, namely: *befriending, planning, confederation* and *coaching* (Spouse 1996, 1998a). These characteristics of effective mentorship relate to Titchen's metaphor of 'critical companionship'. She uses this to describe the professional development role of an expert practitioner when supporting her qualified staff. Titchen identifies three conceptual domains: the *relationship domain*, the *rationality–intuitive domain* and the *facilitative use of self domain* (Titchen 1998). For the purposes of this chapter the categories identified by Spouse from her research into nursing students' professional development will be used. Although the term 'mentor' is used here to describe the relatively short relationship between student and designated staff member, it is being suggested that the same characteristics also apply to relationships between preceptor and new staff member or supervisor and colleague.

Befriending in mentorship

The mentorship relationship appears to be fundamental to learners' eventual survival and success. It is the most complex category, encompassing concepts of befriending and sponsorship. As a result of successful bonding activities and establishment of a secure base, learners engage in clinical practices at different levels of complexity with different types of tuition and support that promote their professional development. In describing this concept from the data, several properties of an effective befriending relationship have been identified as follows.

- Affiliation between learner and mentor based on social interactions initiated by the mentor and designed to promote trust and a sense of warmth and interest. The mentor should be seen as a person through sharing personal feelings and experiences, thus establishing a sense of security for the student
- A secure base from which learners can explore their personal world and the professional world of the clinical setting and to which they can return for support and challenge
- Willingness of the learner to be open and to acknowledge feelings as well as to undertake preparatory work to identify learning needs
- Sponsorship within the clinical team which promotes the learner's personal and professional development within the social and professional context of the placement

Affiliation and a secure base

Affiliation seems to be the key to all the other learning activities in clinical practice. Without effective affiliation learners tend to feel isolated from practice and from the other members of a clinical team. They seem to become invisible, and to be ignored and idle or left to roam the wards looking for something to do or someone to talk to. In many respects the process appears to have characteristics similar to bonding or attachment. Effective mentoring seemed to be like having an attentive host in a foreign culture (which characterised each new placement). It is understandable that newcomers will feel uncomfortable in unfamiliar settings and seek cues to orientate themselves. When considering the different properties of befriending, the importance of the reciprocal nature of the mentor relationship is illustrated by Nicola (Narrative 5.6):

'They (mentors) do end up knowing quite a lot about your worries and how you feel about it all. You have to be honest with them. If you're finding something really hard, then you must say so. The mentor I had most problem with was a very dominant character and I was quite timid and shy and I didn't have the guts to go up to her and say "I want to see you once a week for an hour please. When can we meet?" It was more "I'll wait for her to come and ask me when we can meet". I need to see them to talk over something, or the ability to say "I've had a problem with that. I didn't find it easy, so could we talk through that" or "I've had a really shit day and I need to sit down with you". So you have to communicate quite openly with them and honestly and be assertive about what you want from that relationship. But you have to be prepared to show the vulnerable side of you or stuff you're not finding very easy as well and then hopefully they'll give something back to you. Being accepted as a team member is quite a nice feeling as well. Introducing you to everyone and stuff like that is quite important. I think just being supportive and approachable are key qualities and actually taking time out to sit with someone and say "How was your day?". That's important as well, because that's how you build up trust. And giving encouragement when they've done something good. There's nothing nicer than being praised. It really makes you feel good about it all I think.' (Nicola, interview 11, Narrative 5.6)

Nicola's narrative summarises the experiences of many learners and highlights the importance of a mentor taking the first step in helping newcomers to feel valued and welcome. As Nicola implied, newcomers are expected to expose their vulnerability as learners very early in what is often a short and transitory relationship. Unless there is a similar degree of disclosure from the mentor, the relationship is difficult to develop successfully. In North America, and until recently in the UK, the clinical instructor has been the key informant to learners working and learning in clinical practice. Nursing research into the characteristics of good and bad clinical instructors identified friendliness, honesty, self-confidence, approachability and not belittling learners as highly rated by learners in studies conducted by Mogan & Knox (1987) and Sieh & Bell (1994). The role of a clinical instructor or a nurse teacher who is responsible for several learners allocated to one or more placements tends to be limited and fragmented due to the number of clinical areas that have to be covered. This diminishes the quality of student–teacher relationships and often the teacher's credibility. The functional aspect of a clinical teaching role is like that of the mentor attachment in this study. It would be reasonable to assume that characteristics of good clinical instructors are as relevant in mentoring. Daloz (1986) describes the liberating value of a mentor's acknowledgement of the (adult) learner's personhood and how it promotes creativity and maturation. This is supported by writers from a variety of professional disciplines (Massarik 1979; Oakley 1981; Titchen 1998) and is based on mutual caring and trust which is close to many models used in therapeutic relationships that health care practitioners are encouraged to develop with their patients. The ideal nurse and the ideal mentor have close similarities with the ideal therapist in counselling relationships. Research into effective adult therapeutic relationships substantiates the importance of an empathetic and supportive practitioner (Howe 1993). In this relationship it is only through the development of trust that a client is able to express deeply felt fears and anxieties, to challenge their previously held assumptions and to learn. Child psychologist John Bowlby (1988) describes these characteristics in his attachment theory as central to creating a 'secure base' (Ainsworth *et al.* 1971) and a foundation for relationships from which clients can progress (Bowlby 1988, pp. 137–56). The existence of a client–practitioner bond based on genuine interest and concern, coupled with willingness to be open and human, enables the client to develop feelings of worth and belonging and to explore their emotional world in a way that helps them to interact more successfully with their environment. This seems congruent with mentoring processes that are described by Sally Ballard and Lisa Benrud-Larson in Chapter 3.10. In placements where learners felt attached to their mentor through a secure and supportive relationship, they became confident to participate in clinical practice and to learn from other members of the clinical team. The social and emotional security provided by such caring relationships enabled them to express their worries, fears and learning needs. As a result they were in a position to receive help and to mature both professionally and personally. The feminist sociologist Ann Oakley (1981) found that her research participants related their growth in self-awareness and ability to reflect on their inner world to the quality of their relationship with her.

Effective befriending is particularly important as a lynchpin activity to mentorship and supervision. This is in addition to the sponsorship role provided by the master to his apprentice as described by anthropologist Jean Lave (1991, p. 91). Following effective bonding and sponsorship, students are able to participate effectively within a clinical team. As a result they are given acknowledgement as legitimate members of the community of practitioners. Through the support of a facilitative mentor, it was possible for them to become more self-aware. Not only could they be conscious of their relationships with clients and of their contributions to the overall workload of the setting, but they could also see what was happening in their clinical practice placement and learn. They began to see outside themselves rather than being preoccupied with their internal lives.

Planning

In traditional rural communities learners are assigned to a systematic programme of activities designed to introduce different aspects of the craft. In Jordan's anthropological study of Yucatec Mayan midwives (Jordan 1989), she describes the complexity of their learning processes and its situatedness within the daily life of Yucatec culture. In particular, a midwifery pupil's personal growth and development are considered essential to her acceptance amongst her community of midwives (Jordan 1989, p. 932). She is exposed to a curriculum of professional knowledge that has been handed down from one generation of midwives to the next. Such a curriculum has evolved over time in a stable culture and is part of its fabric. In post-industrialised societies where nurse education has been formalised and regulated, the majority of practical learning takes place in a variety of settings, staffed by transitory teams of practitioners. A formal core curriculum identifies the occupational standards that learners have to achieve before registering to practise. The diversity of clinical settings in which learners are placed necessitates a superimposed, informal curriculum determined by each specific setting. As a result it becomes important for each placement mentor to fuse the formal course requirements and the opportunities that can be provided by the clinical setting with the individual needs of each student. This will depend upon each student's personal course history (the type of placements already experienced and the development of skills and knowledge already achieved) as well as the student's personal inclinations. From the research data, properties of this planning function were identified as follows:

- Providing a menu of experiences available in the clinical area
- Helping the learner to identify areas of the curriculum which are of special relevance
- Helping the learner to organise learning opportunities or to organise visits (to clinics or other departments, etc.)
- Selecting suitable patients (and perhaps members of the clinical team) for the learner to work with and thus to develop identified skills

Students in this study were stimulated and encouraged by mentors willing to help them formulate and achieve their own objectives for the placement. An example of how important is this planning activity is illustrated by Ruth:

'My mentor wants to know about my learning contract from the word go. I liked what I saw of her. I don't feel I'll be staggering around in the dark. Obviously this is my fourth one [learning contract] and I feel a lot happier. I can see what I'm doing and I suppose the module focus gives you a boundary and within that you can build a fence and you can be anywhere in there and you can guide your path through this. They're your guiding light, but within that you can take any path you want and so that's what my personal learning objectives are. That's the path I choose to take as I work through the module. I'm certainly a lot happier about the planning and that will then tell my mentor what I want to get out of my placement with her. When you're working quite closely with someone and she's doing her job of work... I hope to be given a person for myself, not trail after her.' (Ruth, interview 5, Narrative 5.7)

Several educationalists emphasise the benefits of encouraging learners to be autonomous and to follow areas of interest as a means of promoting motivation and effectiveness (Knowles 1975; Rogers 1983). Many mentors find it difficult to anticipate the learning needs of individual students simply because of the complexity of their personal programme pathway. As a result planning has to be a discrete and important part of the mentoring relationship in that it acknowledges the individual needs of each learner so that s/he is not depersonalised (Seed 1991). Rather s/he is recognised as travelling by a unique route through the programme. This activity emulates the ideal and professional relationship with patients that the profession aims to promote (Redfern 1996). Building on learners' earlier experiences and planning a programme of learning that is most relevant to their needs is central to their professional development and provides a good basis for successful induction into the clinical setting (Spouse 1990, p. 21). To be successful, planning requires mentors to have some understanding of the curriculum as it relates to the student's clinical placement, and particularly of the assessment strategy. Coupled with good professional knowledge of their patients or clients and their medical and nursing needs, planning ensures that a good learning experience can be organised. Findings from Australian research of undergraduate nursing learners' clinical experiences (Hart & Rotem 1994) indicate that many staff do not understand learners' needs and do not recognise the necessity to plan their placements. Ideally learners should arrive on their placement having undertaken some preparation, but as Lorna Cowan's example (Chapter 3.3) indicated this does not always happen and may be associated with their level of maturity and stage in their programme. Even when they do come well prepared they will still need their mentors' support and expert local knowledge to adapt their aims to the setting and to find out how they can be achieved. They will also need advice as to which patients and staff members they can work with so they can develop their everyday professional craft knowledge.

Development of clinical skills can take place through a number of media which are similar to those described by Lave as legitimate peripheral participation (Spouse 1998c). Specifically, learners report that they learn through observing staff, by participating in care provision alongside their mentor or another trusted member of staff or by taking responsibility for an increasingly complex case load, commensurate with their ability or just beyond it. Legitimised participation through confederation with an experienced practitioner bears a strong relationship to social learning experienced by humans from childhood. During the process children and adults learn by participating in socially or culturally important activities alongside an experienced practitioner. Socio-cultural theories of learning help to explain development of cognitive and social processes through social interaction and speech (see Spouse 1998b for further discussion of this). Through engagement with their mentors in this manner, students are able to develop their professional skills and their knowledge. This can lead to a sense of personal satisfaction and stimulation to study. To maximise this learning, students need to be given workloads that are planned carefully so that they offer new challenges. They should also be designed to encourage students to rehearse existing skills in unfamiliar contexts and still have the necessary energy to think about the care they are giving and to study it. As identified by the contributors in the subsequent chapters, students also need time that has been planned to discuss their activities with their mentor or with another trusted practitioner. Most learners, in the early stages of their programme particularly, want to practise along-side their mentor. This is an important and continuing strategy to develop necessary attributes and skills. Such a partnership has been called *con-federation* and it symbolises the sponsorship of the newcomer by a member of the community of practice who is willing to share professional knowledge and expertise.

Confederation

Effective confederation takes place when a learner is seen as a full partner, working alongside a mentor. The process should include active partici-pation by the student and a dialogue that explains what is taking place at a level at which the student can understand. From learners' narratives it is clear that this is a crucial element to their success in any clinical placement. It may be assumed that in earlier parts of their course the necessity of this arrangement could be taken for granted as students would possess few clinical skills. By the time they reached the end of their programme many mentors seemed to feel students can manage without this form of support. However, entry to any unfamiliar clinical area presents no less difficult a challenge than those of earlier placements and, not withstanding a mentor's obligation to assess the quality and reliability of learners' practices, the confederate activity provides essential opportunities to learn specialist and expert skills. The nature of confederation is different from the coaching described by Schön (1983) which will be discussed later. The quality of learning gained from confederation can not be achieved if learner and mentor work separately with different patients. It requires mentors to encourage and support learners' participation by constructing a supplementary or peripheral role in providing care. This should take place during any nursing activity such as providing intimate personal care, giving medications, managing a case load of patients or sitting and talking with a patient about his care or with a dying patient and his family. From the data, five specific properties of confederation were identified for this category:

- A trusting relationship between learner and mentor/practitioner exists and the learner is allowed to work in partnership when giving care
- The focus on the activity is mentor initiated and led, in that the mentor identifies nursing actions and carries them out with the learner acting as assistant
- During the activity, the mentor shares her/his craft knowledge about the client's/patient's care needs and the manner in which they are being met. This normally takes place with the mentor articulating thoughts, instincts and knowledge about any observations, processes and procedures as well as conclusions for future action
- The activity may be concerned with any aspect of patient/client care in which mentor and learner are engaged
- The learner is delegated legitimate aspects of patient/client care which contribute to the whole, e.g. contributing to a procedure (such as mobilising a patient) which two nurses can undertake, or discrete tasks commensurate with the level of skill already achieved

During experiences of confederation, learners are able to recognise and learn from their mentor's intuitive or craft knowledge as well as to develop knowledge of how to provide care. This procedural knowledge or script of practice and understanding helps students to develop their understanding of why such care should be provided, and helps them to link their (generalised) classroom learning to what is taking place in practice. Such collaborative activities help learners to develop specific as well as composite skills, to envisage and to engage in the whole process of caregiving and to recognise its component parts as the following narrative by Ruth in her third year as a nursing student indicates. These experiences also help students to develop a range of different approaches to managing similar and different care activities. Often these are retained or remembered in association with particular patients and are stored for future use in similar situations. Such packages of memories of action are known as schemata and form the basis for developing professional craft knowledge (Calderhead 1987, p. 8).

'Their knowledge is a lot greater than mine so I always feel that what they say is a lot more substantiated because of what I've read and the limited experience I've had. So it's nice to hear how they would deal with situations that I've not encountered. Like the lady with the terminal care and how they're dealing with that.' (Ruth, interview 16, Narrative 5.8)

As Ruth identifies, such experiences fuel motivation to explore situations further and encourage her to generate questions and thus to learn. In the process of confederation, students are able to witness how care is planned and provided as a result of observing their mentor's activities of assessing and analysing a patient's needs from moment to moment during the interaction of care giving. This activity requires thoughtful practitioners to review their professional knowledge and to search for relevant schemata for caring for their patients on an individual basis. Thus personal, professional, craft knowledge becomes transformed in to a dynamic and evolutionary reality. Schön (1983) calls this process reflection-in-action and Benner *et al.* (1996) seem to be describing the same sort of activities when they observed expert nurses in action. They call the process of active contemplation whilst in the midst of an activity a state of being present-at-hand. Their study of expert practitioners indicated a similar process of refinement and adjustment of the care-giving activities that personalised schemata of action to specific needs of a client (Benner *et al.* 1996, p. 196). Such practice is highly complex and requires knowledge of a range of sophisticated technical and interpersonal skills as well as an understanding of complex professional knowledge that is often taken for granted. Students exposed to confederation with an experienced practitioner are able to witness such reflection-in-action or being present-at-hand in a manner that is informative and rewarding. An example of this is described by Nicola. She is talking about working with her mentor in the mental health setting:

'Veronica's been really great this term because we'll do something together and she'll turn round and say "What did you think of that?" and I'll tell her how I thought it went and we'll have a discussion about it. She does quite a bit of CBT (cognitive behavioural therapy) work, that's her speciality, so I sat in several times when she's been doing that with a patient and she's been quite good at talking me through what she's doing while she does it. So I suppose I'm learning all the time, but it doesn't seem like learning, it's just like I've opened all my pores up to being receptive to everything that's there. People are just feeding me really with all this knowledge and information.' (Nicola, interview 15, Narrative 5.9)

Such examples describe modes of analysing an operation to achieve specific objectives. Students required a similar but distinct activity that has been labelled 'coaching'. Here learning opportunities continue to be structured by a mentor but the student becomes the key actor in care giving and is supported by the mentor.

Coaching

Several studies indicate that students are frequently left to work alone (Reid 1985; Wilson-Barnett *et al.* 1995; May *et al.* 1997). Whilst this can be rewarding and stimulating for students, its benefits can be made apparent by careful planning. Student and supervisor need opportunities to talk through the planning and implementation of care that is intended to be given, and later what was accomplished. As a result of this combination of preparation, planning, practice and debriefing, students come to develop their self-confidence. They also learn about alternative ways of giving care and about their professional role. Both Ruth's and Nicola's narratives illustrate the importance of this type of relationship with their mentors. Students found it invaluable to have their mentor or a trusted practitioner to tutor them as they led the care giving and to talk them through procedures or to have time to discuss either in advance or afterwards about how to cope with their experiences. These activities are the same as those identified by Sally Ballard (Chapter 3.9) and by Lisa Benrud-Larson (Chapter 3.10) as being so essential to their professional development and which the supervisors in Chapter 3 described in their critical incidents.

Schön (1987) discusses three particular modes of coaching, the *collaborative, follow-me,* and *hall of mirrors.* In case studies of each of these three methods his students presented examples of their skill, using material that could be manipulated until the ideal formula or practice was identified and achieved by the learner (Schön 1987). In the presence of clients or sick patients such practices can be a difficult undertaking in clinical settings. The processes described by Schön are intended to help students learn what good practice feels like, to achieve an effective understanding of skilled performance. This is the same intention as Jordan's description of midwives who use their hands to guide those of their apprentices so that they can learn to know what they were feeling (Jordan 1989). In a similar manner, much of Nicola's (Narrative 5.10) coaching in mental health was concerned with helping her to recognise and acknowledge her own feelings and to work with them so that she could come to understand those of her clients and to learn how best to help them. As with Mary Kavanagh's example (3.5), easy access to a mentor who could both support and challenge her thinking enabled Nicola to share her difficulties and to talk them over and then supplement her ideas through reading and discussions with her peers. Over time and with practice Nicola came to develop a stronger self-image and thus a clearer sense of the boundary between herself and her clients.

'The lady I'd been working with had done quite a lot of self-harm as well. I was amazed because she comes over as a really gentle, timid, meek woman. She's about 30 but looks about 22. So it was quite hard to link the woman who smashed her fists through glass doors with the woman who I was working with. The only problem I had with all of it really was that I came off one shift a bit bemused about my role as a nursing student. I talked this over with M [mentor] later and we discovered it was to do with the patient herself. She has this effect on a lot of people. So it was a bit of a conflict for me and my role. I wouldn't classify myself as a friend of hers, well I am, but a professional friendship somehow. But I was glad to have sorted out my role and making more sense of it. I think working so closely with J and actually being needed by her [are the most significant thing this term]. And being able to contribute something positive to her healing process...You do have to keep a distance from patients on the wards as well... Perhaps that's where it goes back to coping mechanisms and strategies and support systems.' (Nicola, interview 8, Narrative 5.10)

It is possible that Schön's models of coaching which take place away from the real-life environment also have importance to nurse learners as they exemplify a safe place in which to consider practice and could be used to complement activities of the clinical mentor. Certainly such classroom coaching offers students opportunities to develop their knowledge-in-waiting (Spouse 1998b) through scaffolded proleptic instruction from teachers who are well endowed with formal knowledge, and this can be used to supplement students' practical experiences. From the students' data the following properties were identified for the concept of coaching:

- The student is the key actor in a designated nursing activity, rather than the mentor
- Coaching takes place within a supportive relationship where the student is able to respect and trust the mentor's skills (by contrast, when there is a sense of insecurity, comments are viewed as criticism)
- The learning activity is structured to develop the student's knowledge
- The mentor supplements the student's performance by providing specific guidance or information related to the skills practised. These may be procedural or sharing of craft knowledge
- The mentor's dialogue may include questions designed to engage the

student in exploring her/his actions in relation to patient need or to
relevant theory and which challenges the student's perspective

• The mentor provides guidance related to the student's clinical assignment
• Evaluation of performance is discrete, developmental and takes place
away from the patient and should be led by the student

Most students feel acutely self-conscious and worried that they could be
shamed by a mistake and yet need coaching to ensure that they develop
their skills correctly. Unless it was a master class it would have been
unthinkable for Casals to coach his students on the concert platform and
yet students are being exposed to a similar environment by practising on
vulnerable clients. Sloboda identifies five characteristics of a skill: fluency,
rapidity, automaticity, simultaneity and knowledge (Sloboda 1986), none
of which can be effectively developed on an *ad hoc* basis in a public arena
such as the clinical situation unless students have already developed skill
in the basic sequence of activities. This was the difficulty that Barbara
Lovelady's student (3.1) encountered and which is shared by most other
students whose labour is required for the workforce. Schön's students
were already skilled, perhaps at the stage of advanced beginner or beyond
(Dreyfus & Dreyfus 1986). They appeared to be able to operate beyond
close adherence to principles, but had limited ability to discriminate or
implement strategies in response to their perceptions. Through practice
they would have been able to anticipate subsequent moves or problems
and perhaps this could have been better acquired in the privacy of a
practical room or in consultation with their mentor in the manner that
both Sally and Lisa describe. Many nursing activities involve the same
kind of technical dexterity required to play a musical instrument and call
for the level of proficiency identified by Sloboda (1986) before they can be
overlaid with additional activities (simultaneity) that are associated with
professional practice. Additional activities include knowing how to
respond to a suicidal client, how to reassure a patient whilst undertaking a
sensitive assessment of his needs in a complex situation, or how to use
awareness of a need to bring formal know-how into use. From an
extensive review of the literature, Ericsson and his colleagues found that
undertaking complex skills requires repeated exposure and feedback to
enable practitioners to improve their performance, and that ten years was
the average time it took to become expert (Ericsson *et al.* 1993). The ideal
role of coach is to facilitate this analysis of experience by creating time for
students to discuss their practice as well as to identify opportunities that
expose them to increasingly complex versions of an activity that will
develop their competence further.

Sally's narrative of being prepared to admit a patient on her own provides an example of how she was supported in developing her professional knowledge and her self-confidence. In a similar situation Lisa had been given a patient who challenged her professional knowledge. With her mentor's support Lisa was able to critically examine what had taken place and to learn from the experience whilst also developing her self-confidence. Part of such discussions should help students to identify key characteristics of the client's care that may be found to be problematic so that students can more easily anticipate them in future. Experience of being assigned a caseload and having a trusted mentor as a secure base to return to for support is important. Sharing experiences, discussing them and considering the mentor's ideas and questions stimulate students to consider alternative perspectives, to read around the pathology and therapeutic aspects of their patient's condition and to try out new practices. In a similar but more complex way, Claire-Louise Hatton's narrative (Chapter 3.7) of how she tried to introduce the important concept of professional artistry into her student's practice indicates the delicacy of professional development and the supervisor's role. Her observations are not unique to students and can just as easily apply to experienced colleagues (as Maggie's narrative indicated, 5.1). A mentor's investment of trust and respect in the learner increases self-confidence and thus increases motivation. The scaffolded activity encouraging both discussion between learner and mentor about the issues (*intermental* activity: Vygotsky 1978) and personal reflection and analysis (*intramental* activity) helps learners to develop professional knowledge more effectively than if they have been left to get on or to muddle through with the caregiving alone. Such experiences promote and refine the acquisition of new language to describe professional activities as well as to develop new insights. Examples of students' accounts of good mentorship demonstrate that confidence in their mentor coupled with increasing understanding helps students to construct questions that extend their understanding and thus their practical knowledge (increasing their zone of proximal development: Palincsar 1986). These examples (Chapters 3.9, 3.10) seem to correlate with a concept that, through scaffolded activity, learners began to develop their own knowledge base for practice and to develop schema that inform their future actions. Rogoff argues that this appropriation of knowledge is more than simply internalisation or translation of information from an external to an internal source (Rogoff 1995). She argues that through participation in a dialogue with an experienced practitioner, knowledge and action become integral, rather like parts of a hologram where each aspect contains the whole. This seems more than the development of Schön's knowing-in-action, which is related to expertise rather than development of expertise. Both Rogoff's and Schön's concepts of inherent knowledge in action suggest that the process is smooth and unproblematic. Learner experiences suggest that this may be the case when they have accumulated sufficient scripts to be able to operate with confidence, in the routine and ready-to-hand mode of using tacit knowledge that requires no consideration. The learning environment between learner and mentor match the sort of relationship advocated by Daloz (1986), a relationship in which support and challenge are high and where threat is absent. Such an environment allows learners to extend their personal and professional knowledge as well as to be given a vision for future development.

By contrast, on occasions when students feel insufficiently supported or befriended by their supervisors, they feel inhibited to ask questions in case these are interpreted as a challenge to their mentor's practice, as Ruth describes below in Narrative 5.11:

'You've got to be diplomatic really, not deliberately antagonise people. That's quite difficult if you've got to challenge people. It's a personality thing. My mentor is great if I say "Can you tell me why you did that?" or "Why should I be doing that?" and she can back it up and not be angry about it. I can well see other members of staff getting quite defensive about the way things are done... I think you have to play it by ear... but you've got to be humble and get on with them and you have to feel your way into the relationship... My mentor did say to me that she wanted me to say if I had any problems and be honest with her. I'm not sure I could be totally honest, but I feel I could say things if I wanted to.' (Ruth interview 12, Narrative 5.11)

A number of writers have identified that in many situations it is considered to be bad manners or too challenging to ask questions of a more senior person. This perception seems to be supported by studies of apprenticeship relationships, in particular the findings of Goody and her colleagues. Goody (1978) came to the conclusion that questioning depended upon a sophisticated hierarchy of relationships. It was considered inappropriate for apprentices to ask questions of their own master but legitimate to ask another senior member of the community. It would seem that for students to feel safe to ask questions it is necessary for their mentor to be willing to give up her authority and to become a professional friend, thus minimising any fear of threat (Rogers 1983). In other settings, hearing a mentor question her own practice provides students with a formula for asking their own questions. Lorna's narrative (Chapter 3.3) indicates that not all mentors feel sufficiently confident about their own practice to accept questioning as curiosity rather than as criticism. Being able to talk about personal practice in a critical manner requires a great deal of skill and security in their role. Contributing to such a sense of security is the warmth and respect that can be developed between mentor and student. Only under such conditions can students feel safe within their new community and have the confidence to ask questions.

As in the confederate activity, the experiences that students enjoyed when being coached by their mentor demonstrate the importance of interpersonal dialogue as a means to reformulate their thinking about practice. In many instances students framed questions evolving from their observations and any consequent dissonance that they experienced. Confederate and coaching activities are important for students whilst they lack relevant skills and knowledge for the clinical placement. Once mentors believe that students are safe to practise alone, it is important to give them opportunities to consolidate and develop their learning further by working on their own, knowing that if necessary an experienced team member can provide support.

The four important components of the mentor/supervisor role, befriending, planning, confederacy and coaching, have relevance for any new practitioner to a clinical setting irrespective of whether the practitioner is a student or an experienced professional. In the early weeks of their orientation to unfamiliar practice settings, newcomers need sponsorship to their new community of practice by someone who is willing to befriend them and to help them assess and plan strategies to meet their learning needs. Collaborative activities of confederation and coaching can provide the much needed support which promotes and ensures that students and staff can work as learners when confronted with unfamiliar situations and experiences.

References

Ainsworth, M. D. S., Bell, S. M. & Stayton, D. J. (1971) Individual differences in strange situation behaviour of one year olds. In *The Origins of Human Social Relations* H. R. Schaffer (ed.), pp. 15–57. Academic Press, London.

Bandura, A. (1977) *Social Learning Theory*. Prentice Hall, New Jersey.

Benner, P., Tanner, C.A. & Chesla, C.A. (eds) (1996) *Expertise in Nursing Practice: Caring, Clinical Judgement and Ethics*. Springer, Cambridge, Mass.

Bowlby, J. (1988) *A Secure Base: Clinical Application of Attachment Theory*. Routledge, London.

Brim, O. G. & Wheeler, S. (1966) *Socialization after Childhood: Two Essays*. John Wiley, New York.

Brown, S. & McIntyre, D. (1993) *Making Sense of Teaching*. Open University Press, Buckingham.

Bruner, J. (1986) *Actual Minds, Possible Worlds*. Harvard University Press, Cambridge, Mass.

Calderhead, J. (1987) *Exploring Teachers' Thinking*. Cassell Education, London.

Conrad, L. & Phillips, E. M. (1995) From isolation to collaboration: a positive change for postgraduate women? *Higher Education* **30** (3), 313–22.

Daloz, L. A. (1986) *Effective Teaching and Mentoring.* Jossey Bass, San Francisco.

Dreyfus, H. L. & Dreyfus, S. E. (1986) *Mind Over Machine: The Power of Human Intuition and Expertise in the Era of the Computer.* Basil Blackwell, Oxford.

Ericsson, K.A., Krampe, R. Th. & Tesch-Römer, C. (1993) The role of deliberate practice in the acquisition of expert performance. *Psychological Review* **100** (3), 363–406.

Glazer, M. (1982) The threat of the stranger: vulnerability, reciprocity and field-work. In *The Ethics of Social Research: Fieldwork Regulation and Publication* (J. Sieber, ed.), pp. 49–70. Springer Verlag, New York.

Goody, E. N. (1978) Toward a theory of questions. In *Questions and Politeness: Strategies in Social Interaction* (E.N. Goody, ed.), pp. 17–43. Cambridge University Press, Cambridge.

Hallsdórsdóttir, S. (1989) The essential structure of a caring and uncaring encounter with a teacher: The perspective of the nursing student. In *The Caring Imperative in Education* (M. Leininger & J. Watson, eds), pp. 95–108. National League for Nursing, New York. 1990.

Hart, G. & Rotem, A. (1994) The best and worst: students' experiences of clinical education. *Australian Journal of Advanced Nursing* **12** (3), March-May, pp. 26–33.

Howe, D. (1993) *On Being a Client: Understanding the Process of Counselling and Psychotherapy.* Sage Publications, London.

Ingleton, C. (1995) Gender and learning: does emotion make a difference? *Higher Education* **30** (3), 323–35.

Jordan, B. (1989) Cosmopolitical obstetrics: some insights from the training of traditional midwives. *Social Science and Medicine* **28** (9), 925–44.

Knowles, M. (1975) *The Adult Learner: A Neglected Species*, 4th edn Gulf Publishing, Houston.

Lave, J. (1991) Situating learning in communities of practice. In *Perspectives on Social Shared Cognition* (L. B. Resnick, J. M. Levine & S. D. Teasley, eds), pp. 63–82. American Psychological Association, Washington, DC.

Masserik, F. (1979) The interviewing process re-examined. In *Human Inquiry* (P. Reason & J. Rowan, eds), pp. 201–6. John Wiley, Chichester.

May, N., Veitch, L., McIntosh, J. B. & Alexander, M. F. (1997) Preparation for Practice: Evaluation of Nurse and Midwife Education in Scotland, 1992 Programmes. Department of Nursing and Community Health, Glasgow Caledonian University. Funded by the National Board for Nursing, Midwifery and Health Visiting for Scotland.

Mead, G. H. (1934) *Mind, Self and Society.* University of Chicago Press, Chicago.

Mogan, L. & Knox, J. (1987) Characteristics of 'best' and 'worst' clinical teachers as perceived by university faculty and students. *Journal of Advanced Nursing* **12** 331–7.

Nicholson, N. (1987) Work role transitions: progress and outcomes. In *Psychology at Work* 3rd edn (P. Warr, ed.), pp. 160–77. Penguin Books, Harmondsworth.

Oakley, A. (1981) Interviewing women: a contradiction in terms. In *Doing Feminist Research* (H. Roberts, ed.). Routledge, London.

Palinesar, A. S. (1986) The role of dialogue in scaffolded instruction. *Educational Psychologist* **21** (1 and 2), 73–98.

Redfern, S. (1996) Individualised patient care: its meaning and practice in a general setting. *Nursing Times Research* **1** (1), 22–33.

Reid, N. G. (1985) The effective training of nurses: manpower implications *International Journal of Nursing Studies* **22** (2), 89–98.

Rogers, C. (1983) *Freedom to Learn for the 80s*. Merrill, New York.

Rogoff, B. (1990) *Apprenticeship in Thinking: Cognitive Development in Social Context*. Oxford University Press, New York.

Rogoff, B. (1995) Observing sociocultural activity on three planes: participatory appropriation, guided participation and apprenticeship. In *Sociocultural Studies of the Mind* (J. V. Wertsch, P. Del Rio & A. Alvarez, eds), pp. 139–63. Cambridge University Press, Cambridge.

Schön, D. (1983) *The Reflective Practitioner : How Professionals Think in Action*. Ashgate, Aldershot.

Schön, D. (1987) *Educating the Reflective Practitioner. Toward a New Design for Teaching and Learning in the Professions*. Jossey Bass, San Francisco.

Seed, A. (1991) Becoming a registered nurse – the students' perspective. A longitudinal qualitative analysis of the emergent views of a cohort of student nurses during their 3 year training for general registration. Leeds Polytechnic and CNAA, unpublished DPhil.

Sieh, S. & Bell, S. K. (1994) Perceptions of effective clinical teachers in Associate degree programs. *Journal of Nursing Education* **33** (9), 389–94.

Sloboda, J. (1986) What is skill and how is it acquired? In *Learning Through Life, 1 : Culture and Processes of Adult Learning. A Reader* (M. Thorpe, R. Edwards & A. Hanson, eds), pp. 253–73. Routledge in association with The Open University, 1993

Spouse, J. (1990) *An Ethos for Learning* Scutari Press, London.

Spouse, J. (1996) The effective mentor: a model for student learning in clinical practice. *Nursing Times Research* **1** (2), 120–33.

Spouse, J. (1998a) Understanding learning in the professional context: Five case studies of nurses from a pre-registration degree programme. Unpublished PhD thesis, University of Bath.

Spouse, J. (1998b) Scaffolding student learning clinical practice. *Nurse Education Today* **18**, 259–66.

Spouse, J. (1998c) Learning to nurse through legitimate peripheral participation. *Nurse Education Today* **18**, 345–51.

Titchen, A. (1998) A Conceptual Framework for Facilitating Learning in Clinical Practice. Occasional Paper No. 2, Radcliffe Infirmary, Oxford, Royal College of Nursing Institute.

van Maanen, J. (1976) Breaking in: socialization to work. In *Handbook of Work Organization and Society* (R. Dubin, ed.), pp. 67–130. Rand McNally College Publication Co., Chicago.

van Maanen, J. (ed.) (1977) Introduction: the promise of career studies. In

Organizational Careers: Some New Perspectives, pp. 1–13. John Wiley, London.

Vygotsky, L. S. (1978) *Mind in society: The development of higher psychological processes* (M. Cole, V. J. Steiner, S. Scribner & E. Suberman, eds). Harvard University Press, Cambridge, Mass.

Wax, R. H. (1952) Field methods and techniques: reciprocity as a field technique. *Human Organization* **11**, 32–7.

Wilson-Barnett, J., Butterworth, T., White, E., Twinn, S., Davies, S. & Riley, L. (1995) Clinical support and the Project 2000 nursing student: factors influencing this process. *Journal of Advanced Nursing* **21**, 1152–8.

Wiseman, R. (1994) Role model behaviours in the clinical setting. *Journal of Nursing Education* **33** (9), 405–10.

Chapter 6

Supervision in Professional Practice: Implications for Educationalists and Practitioners

Jenny Spouse

What kinds of knowledge do supervisors need to develop in order to be effective in their role? How can these be developed or imparted to clinicians? What models of practice can be used to support their development? These are important questions that this chapter will address. It builds on the earlier case studies to examine how effective supervision may be developed in clinical settings. Detailed information about the process of supervision is brought to life by vivid individual critical incidents described by the ten practitioners. They demonstrate the complexity of the supervisory relationship. Processes that are engaged need to be thought about carefully, and these critical incidents highlight some of the considerations and practices that help to inform good practice. These practitioners were working in settings where professional supervision was becoming an accepted part of professional life. In settings in which supervision is not an identified and resourced activity, accounts could be very different. Rudd and Wolsey in Chapter 4.2 provide information about the specification of supervision and use of resources when developing and implementing such supervisory structures in one nursing service. Their considerations of structural issues influencing professional supervision are the foundation for future successful development, especially if it is going to be adopted throughout a service. The case study of experienced practitioners working in unfamiliar settings (Davies, Simic and Gregson, Chapter 4.1) gives some ideas about how discussions within supervision may change over time and as participants develop their identity within their relationship and the organisation.

In his exploration of a range of models and purposes of supervision (Chapter 2), Northcott identifies the distinction between appraisal and supervision. He examines the relationship between the two processes and considers how each activity can contribute to personal development when conducted in a supportive environment. Chapter 2 provides a model which may be used to structure some supervisory relationships where close partnerships are useful in developing personal practice. This model has relevance across all settings but provides little information about how to prepare staff to undertake such activities. There is also an implicit assumption that supervision will only work as a one-to-one partnership. Whilst this provides a model for many situations and thus interactions, there are other approaches that can be used as well. Possibly the most challenging, supportive and even economical (in some settings) of these approaches is through participation in action learning circles among peers who are supported by a facilitator. Such an approach provides a powerful way for groups of practitioners to explore their practice, to share their experiences and to learn new ways of operating through exchanges of narratives. Perhaps because health care practitioners are concerned with human experiences they become particularly adept at listening to their patients' or clients' accounts and also enjoy sharing their own accounts of experience. Indeed it would seem that many students rely upon such exchanges to develop their own professional knowledge (Spouse 1998a). Several writers recognise the importance of story telling or exchanges of narratives as a means of sharing specialist knowledge that is concerned with everyday living rather than with the formal (textbook) knowledge that has been abstracted and refined from practice and generalised. This sharing of craft knowledge or folk knowledge (Bruner 1986) provides a fundamental resource for everyday existence. It relies on good communication systems within organisations to ensure that practices are shared and developed. Sometimes such craft knowledge can perpetuate unsatisfactory practices and thus practitioners need the stimulus of a critical approach which is supported by careful documentation and evaluation, to allow progress to be achieved. Revans' work in hospital settings led him to conclude that collaborative activities among peers and shared problem solving helped to promote team work as well as to encourage self-confidence and improved problem solving skills (Revans 1982). Both these approaches of one-to-one and group activities can foster such skills whilst providing effective professional development. Both encourage attitudes of critical inquiry and reflective practice. Setting up programmes which encourage such approaches is perhaps the most important stage in the whole process. In this chapter I will explore the approaches I used in a 10-week part-time academic course to prepare health care practitioners for their supervisory role in relation to both colleagues and students.

The course

The 150-hour course was offered at two academic levels (undergraduate level 2/3 and postgraduate level) with groups of students who studied separately over 10 or 12 weeks respectively and a total of 35 hours' attendance in the university. Students undertaking the undergraduate module were either studying it as a stand-alone unit or as part of a modular degree programme. The postgraduate module was taken as a single-module short course. Many of the students had not studied for some time and needed encouragement and time to redevelop their academic skills. Most of the students were women with families, working full time whilst studying in their own time. This meant that they were experiencing a great deal of pressure, requiring careful planning so that they could cope with all the various demands upon their time. Many were returning to part-time study with many years of experience as highly competent practitioners but held a poor self-image of themselves as learners. They saw undertaking an undergraduate degree as a potential threat to their self-esteem. The challenge of facing unfamiliar material after many years of consolidation of existing knowledge can be painful. It may take students some time to appreciate that it is not a failure of self, but simply the experience of encountering unfamiliar ideas and approaches that have to be recognised and learned (Taylor 1987). Taylor provides a useful model to describe the stages through which learners progress when encountering such experiences, and her ideas were used as much as possible to structure the course. The programme was based on an experiential model and students were asked to bring examples from their own practice or experience with which to work. Many had worked with students, some with colleagues, but all had knowledge of being supervised. They had a wealth of experiences to use as a basis for their own learning. Experiential learning assumes that students are more able to benefit from learning through their own experiences and from engaging in a process of reflection, analysis and study of any issues that are of particular interest. Reflection may be a difficult activity to undertake alone and the course was designed to encourage students to feel sufficiently confident to share experiences with their peers. This made it important to develop a relaxed and friendly atmosphere to the sessions. It also meant that as the teacher I had to adopt a facilitative approach to promoting learning rather than feel that I had to have all the ideas and answers. It did not mean that I could rely upon the students to do all the work, and a proportion of theoretical material was introduced to stimulate discussion, insight and development. Before starting the course, students were provided with a handbook detailing the module learning outcomes and the nature of the learning activities of their programme. It also contained a copy of the course criteria used to assess academic work, some (helpful) tips about the module and a reading list. The two latter items were generated from past students' recommendations and evaluation comments on the module. A preliminary timetable indicated the weekly topic areas that could be addressed but was also identified as a means of providing a framework for further negotiation by the students. This timetable included several sessions that were 'empty' and would be negotiated with them. Students were encouraged to work as partners in their learning and to develop co-operative strategies that allowed them to benefit from each others' knowledge. The educational process was designed to mimic and encourage investigative activity that it was hoped participants (the students) would use in their supervisory relationships and which would help them to develop the necessary skills of co-operative dialogue and problem solving. In essence they would be developing a repertoire of supervisory skills that they had examined critically over the term. Providing theoretical information would help them to find ways in which their activities could be explained and justified. These approaches were developed with a commitment to supporting learners to feel responsible for their own learning and to give them opportunities to investigate issues that were important to them. This encourages them to take a deep approach to their learning which is more meaningful and relevant to their everyday practice (Marton & Säljö 1997). Abercrombie's work of promoting learning through group interaction provided further evidence of the value of such approaches that was reinforced by research into social learning activities in humans (Abercrombie 1969; Wertsch & Stone 1979; Brown *et al.* 1989; Benner *et al.* 1996; Spouse 1998b).

Learning and teaching activities

In the first session of the programme students were encouraged to develop a definition of supervision for themselves and to discuss this in pairs. Artefacts such as pictures and wooden or stone sculptures were used as a medium through which students could trigger their thinking. The artwork either came from books of art that I personally found attractive, or objects that I had acquired on my travels. They had not been specifically chosen because of any overt relationship with the course. Over several years I have become delighted and intrigued at the different ways in which the same images elicit a variety of views from participants. Students were then encouraged to share their views in a larger group, usually no more than six people, and to determine their hopes and expectations of the course. From these small group discussions we then developed a statement of their aims and objectives for the module and the topic areas that they wished to explore. This collaborative approach to designing the course-in-action encouraged students to take responsibility for the sessions and to become actively involved in their own learning. It set the scene for the approaches to learning that are used over the term and helped students to develop social and emotional ties with each other. They came to learn about each other's perceptions of the course and the levels of understanding that existed. This helped to brush away many of the anxieties that herald the first days of a course.

Three key activities were used throughout the course to promote learning. Students were encouraged to develop a contract of their own learning intentions based on those of the course but focused on a particular aspect of their own interest. Each student worked over the first seven weeks of the ten-week programme to develop and to refine a learning contract. The second activity was through analysis and discussion of a critical incident from their own experience which students were encouraged to share in their base group or action learning group of five or six other colleagues. The third key activity was to encourage students to learn through writing, by documenting their experiences in a private journal or diary and through their assignments. Apart from their summative or final assignment for the module of learning, this documentation did not necessarily have to be totally through writing. Students were encouraged to use art as a medium of expression, either through painting or drawing or through collecting images which represented their conceptualisation of supervision and the area of supervision in which they were particularly interested. Each of these areas of learning will now be explored more fully.

Using a learning contract

Learning contracts have been a familiar device in nurse education for some years (Tompkins & McGraw 1981; Burns 1992; Jarvis & Gibson 1997) and are often based on a framework devised by the American adult educator, Malcolm Knowles (1975). Working with a philosophy of student empowerment and autonomy, students are encouraged to identify their own learning needs; to design a strategy by which the needs can be met; and to describe the evidence they would provide to demonstrate achievement of their learning intentions. They are also expected to identify suitable criteria that would define the quality of the work. It was not intended that learning contracts would become a tight straitjacket, confining students to a particular course of action. They would be both a tool for helping them learn and a tool to develop a product of their learning. As students became more familiar with their subject and more able to find ways in which they could talk about the issues with which they were concerned, so they were able to be more specific and focused on what they wished to examine. Such development took place over most of the module and could not be achieved within the first few weeks. Personal learning contracts were developed over a cycle of writing, discussion both with their peers and with me as their teacher, and re-writing, until everyone felt satisfied that they represented both what was desired and what was achievable within the time frame. Most of this discussion took place within base peer groups. A 30-minute tutorial slot was also included within the module plan for each student. Inevitably students' learning needs vary and such time slots are rarely sufficient to meet the needs of all the students.

Learning through documentation

Documentation of understanding is a powerful way to develop personal thought and understanding (Allen *et al.* 1989). Most usually documentation is achieved through writing, particularly in the form of assignments. But this approach assumes a high level of competency in writing which can be achieved only over a long period of time and practice. Such achievement is closely associated with self-confidence and not everyone is good at expressing personal and tentative thoughts through words. Neil Fleming's work supplementing use of reading and writing with auditory, kinaesthetic and visual modes of learning provides a valuable basis for offering students alternative media for these first tentative steps of understanding (Fleming 1995). All these approaches were incorporated into the learning processes used in the module.

In assuming that students were engaged in some form of supervisory relationship during the course, they were encouraged to keep a record of their experiences in the form of a journal (Holly 1989). This was intended to provide a log of their experiences which they could return to when deciding upon the purpose and focus of their assignment. It also provided an opportunity to think about practical issues which could have been lost without some form of personal record keeping. By engaging in keeping a journal, students were in a better position to discover questions that needed answering and thus to recognise the boundaries of their own knowledge (Hedlund *et al.* 1989). If students chose to share these experiences, they could then be explored further with their base group of peers. The personal element of their experiences was valued and students were encouraged to consider the affective or emotional aspects so that they could increase their own understanding of what was taking place for them as well as for their supervisory colleague (Boud *et al.* 1985). Not all students chose to use this strategy and at the end of the course several recognised that they would have been much more focused and thus able to gain more support when engaged in their base group presentation and discussion if they had undertaken some preliminary preparation.

Using visualisation to support students' learning was undertaken through two particular forms: diagramming and artwork. The teaching sessions provided a diagrammatic representation of the material and students were encouraged to develop their own whenever undertaking reading or in preparation for their presentation. Some students chose to develop schema of their experiences through diagramming in their journals. In addition they were encouraged to create diagrams or spider-grams summarising their understanding. These could provide a visual image of the relationship between different aspects of their understanding of the topic. Entwistle describes this process of refinement and structuring of knowledge as development of a knowledge object (Entwistle 1998). Such a technique may be used in a number of ways: whilst reading articles, during and following presentations of formal material or to summarise base group discussions. This process of schematising thinking and learn-ing provided a useful means for creating accessible summaries and links between course material and personal practice. The process of analysis, condensation of material into a diagrammatic model based on a metaphor from the students' visualisation of the topic, required them to take a deep approach to their learning. A second strategy, derived from the same principles, was to encourage students to value their intuition and pre-conscious understandings of their supervisory roles through creating artwork. Creating images often assists in tapping into the pre-conscious, and has been used extensively in art therapy and in schools and more recently as a medium for data collection (see Spouse 1998a, pp. 94–9). This was achieved in two different ways. With some groups, students were supplied with paper and a variety of colouring materials, crayons, chalks, pens, water-based paint and a range of brushes and sponges with which to make their mark. Inevitably most students had not practised any form of creative drawing since they were in school and they were concerned that their attempts could be ridiculed as being childish. This fear was acknowledged and they were reassured that it was not the art product that was of importance but the discourse they would enter into during its creation and when discussing their work with a colleague. To further reassure them I also entered into the activity, also feeling vulnerable due to my own incompetence in art. A more structured version of this approach was used for the undergraduate course. Students were encouraged to undertake the same type of activity for their first assignment of the module by creating a pictorial definition of supervision. The results were extra-ordinarily creative and exciting. Some chose to create a collage of mate-rials (silver paper, magazine pictures, etc.) whilst others used paint, crayon or chalk. To support their images, students were required to write a 500-word rationale for their work. This ensured that their message could be clearly understood. Both aspects of their work contributed to their assignment. In preparation for this assessment activity, students were asked to decide upon the criteria that should be used to assess their work. These were based on the course criteria but applied to the artwork. A fundamental criterion for success was the ability to express the core functions of the supervisory process. In both activities the results were enthralling, giving wonderful opportunities for fruitful discussion and development of new understandings. Their group discussions and the subsequent decision-making process gave students an opportunity to study the criteria in depth and to clarify their understanding of the skills they were being asked to demonstrate. In essence they were becoming more fully acquainted with the academic standards of the course.

Learning through group work

Throughout the term students were encouraged to share any of their journal or assignment work with their base group peers. This encouraged dialogue between their work and their thinking, which introduced a range of perspectives, not only on their work but also to their understanding of supervisory activities. In the process they shared their literature resources and debated their meaning, thus refining their thinking and developing their ability to think critically about issues which were important to them. They also developed their group working and interpersonal skills and gained self-confidence and self-discipline. In essence the activities helped students to develop their professional skills and provided a lived experience of peer supervision. It was anticipated that students would be able to use such skills in their own clinical setting, either to support their colleagues in supervisory relationships on a one-to-one basis or as a member of a group. These activities were developed through action learning circles, a strategy designed to encourage co-operative learning and problem solving. Central to the process is the ability of participants to problematise their work and to explore critical incidents that they had encountered in their practice.

Identifying a critical incident

Motivation to learn often arises from seemingly trivial events which have got under our skin. Frequently they can go unnoticed at a conscious level but they nag away at us until we are able to recognise what is causing the problem. On other occasions we are faced with a dilemma which dominates our thinking and it is only through sharing that it can be unravelled. These situations can be described as critical incidents. Such experiences cause some pause for thought or, as Boyd & Fales (1983) identify, 'inner discomfort'. Through the unravelling process, the incidents can be examined more critically and successfully. This process is called problematising and encourages a more objective view to be taken. Critical incidents were first identified by Flanagan (1954) as a strategy to improve a teaching programme for airline pilots. To train and assess pilots effectively they needed to know what constituted best practice. Pilots were asked to describe situations that they commonly faced and how they dealt with them. Critical incidents have been used throughout the world since then to identify standards of performance as well as to support problem solving. In nursing they were first reported to be used to heighten students' awareness of what they were encountering in practice and to help them develop the necessary language to talk about their experiences (Clamp 1980). This complexity of health care activities requires careful consideration of each of the several components and is a valuable means to identifying key issues. Re-examining the experience or reflecting about it permits new insights to be developed as well as motivating further inquiry to supplement existing knowledge. Students were encouraged to use a structure from one of the several models of reflection which were offered to them. A simple framework is to describe 'What I did; what happened; what was different from what I expected; what I did not do; why and what I did instead; so what now: what can I learn?' Providing participants of the action learning group felt confident that they would not be judged or criticised, the detail of their discussion often depended upon their ability to delve at a deep level into what took place and to acknowledge their own accompanying feelings. This sort of analysis is made easier with a more structured model such as those offered by Jack Mezirow (1981) or David Tripp (1993) which provide critical questions to ask oneself in preparation for the presentation and can enable a richer experience during the action learning circle presentation. Feelings were an important aspect of the debriefing process and frequently it was not until they had been recognised and shared by the presenter that effective learning could be undertaken (Boud 1985). Most people try to process a complex and large event which often needs to be reduced to its smaller key components. It is this process which is often made easier by working in an action learning circle.

Setting up action learning circles

The underlying belief of action learning circles is that individuals normally work better in groups and are capable of resolving their own problems. They need to be given the opportunity to work towards solutions in a supportive and constructive environment; to be given different perspectives with which to reframe their reality and thus to problem solve. This approach could only be successful if students were willing to work together and to share their thoughts and feelings. Without this climate of trust and openness, discussions tended to be at a superficial level concerned with exchanges of factual information and often punctuated by long silences. This finding is supported by Miller when researching pre-registration education and use of reflective practice in classroom activities (Miller 1995). Towards developing a climate of trust, students were encouraged to create a peer base group of five or six students for themselves in the first session of the module and to work within that group to create a trusting environment. This was promoted by initial teaching activities which included asking each base group to develop and agree their own ground rules of structure and function. They were also asked to decide upon a strategy that would ensure each member had an opportunity to present and analyse their own critical incident, to facilitate another member's presentation and to act as supporter for their peers.

For success this requires a commitment from each member of the circle to:

- Attend regularly and negotiate with the group members for anticipated absence
- Be willing to be open and honest about one's own feelings of success and failure
- Listen actively to the presenter's story and support her/him in finding a solution which meets personal need

These three functions were important to develop a democratic climate within each group and for students to develop effective skills in presenting information, listening to others and formulating questions which supported their colleagues' analytical and reflective skills. Figure 6.1 gives a model of the skills and activities that may be developed when working in an action learning circle.

How does an action learning circle work?

Several models of functioning in an action learning circle were used by the students depending upon their group's preference. The key function is to provide opportunities for each member to take turns to present and solve a problem within the group circle. This can be achieved by each session being devoted to only one presenter or to two or three. Much depends upon the amount of time that is available for the activity. In the module, the action learning circles were the last part of the three-hour session and

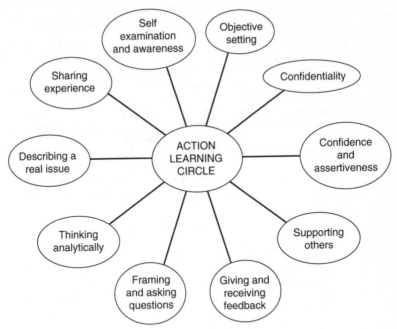

Fig. 6.1   The skills and processes that are involved in action learning circles.

were of one and a quarter hours duration. Several groups chose to have two or three presentations each week, requiring careful time keeping to ensure that each presenter had a fair share of the time. Other groups chose to use an approach whereby each week every member was invited to say whether there was an issue that was concerning them. The group then decided whether there were any common features and then worked through these together. This meant that each member had the opportunity to present a brief summary of the key features of their issue every week. The group then worked collaboratively to examine the key issues. A third approach was for a different circle member to make a presentation at each meeting and to work through the cycle.

Whichever model was used, groups often found that an issue surfaced which was common to several members. The weekly meetings meant that members could also give feedback on the progress of their action plans. It was essential to the success of each action learning circle that the group identified for each meeting a member who would take responsibility for ensuring that all members carried out the process correctly. This would have to be clarified by the ground rules for the group and could include sentences that had been agreed for use, such as to stop someone giving advice or talking too much in an unfocused manner. Specific roles for each group member are identified in Fig. 6.2.

Time in the session	Facilitator's role	Presenter's role	Supporter's role
Beginning	Re-establishing the agreed ground rules for the group; checking the time allocation; checking the agreed procedure for the session	Describing the critical incident and taking ownership of the issues Often this is made easier if presenters have first written this out in their journal and have begun to order the information and to develop their understanding	Observing the presenter's body language; listening to the narrative and listening for what may have been omitted. Considering the implications of the issues for the presenter and those associated with it
Middle	Ensuring that no one person dominates the presenter; the presenter follows the analytical framework of description, analysis and action planning as far as possible	Exploring the critical incident by responding to questions and following through ideas that have been stimulated by the questions (This is often difficult to do if many questions are asked rapidly and can be made easier if the session is tape-recorded for private listening later)	Framing questions designed: to test own understanding of the problem; to probe for the wider implications of the issue; to explore any underlying causes/ issues; to promote analytical thinking; to reflect back to the presenter what has been said for reconsideration
End	Ensuring that time boundaries are observed; checking that the group members are aware of their role. Summarises the discussion for the presenter. Invites the presenter's permission for the group to give feedback, which does not need to be acknowledged	Ventilating feelings associated with the issue, this makes it much easier to see the situation clearly Exploring future actions. Asking 'What if' questions, specifying particular points	Accepting and acknowledging the presenter's feelings. Encouraging the presenter to work through the possible consequences of proposed actions by asking questions. Sometimes the presenter may ask for ideas, but these should only be offered at the end of the session when s/he has exhausted any personal solutions

Fig. 6.2   The role of the action learning circle members.

Over the term students became more confident in their group and were able to develop both their presentation and their listening abilities. One term is a very short time in which to become skilled in participating in such activities but they did provide an experience which students could take back and use in their own clinical setting. Some groups met outside the academic time and were able to develop stronger relationships that could sustain them through more challenging settings. The long-term benefits of these processes are difficult to assert. In their evaluations most participants stated that their self-confidence had grown and that they felt more able to seek help. They also believed that they had a greater understanding of how to support students or colleagues. By engaging wholeheartedly in a discourse about their practice, students were able to take a more critical approach to many taken-for-granted issues and to find ways of making improvements.

References

Abercrombie, M.L.J. (1969) *The Anatomy of Judgement*. Penguin, Harmondsworth.

Allen, D.G., Bowers, B. & Diekelman, N. (1989) Writing to learn: A reconceptualization of thinking and writing in the nursing curriculum. *Journal of Nursing Education* **28** (1), 6–11.

Benner, P., Tanner, C. A. & Chesla, C. A. (1996) *Expertise in Nursing Practice: Caring, Clinical Judgement and Ethics*. Springer, Cambridge, Mass.

Boud, D., Keogh, R. & Walker, D. (1985) *Reflection: Turning Experience into Learning*. Kogan Page, London.

Boyd, E. M. Fales, A. W. (1983) Reflective learning: key to learning from experience. *Journal of Humanistic Psychology* **23** (2), 99–117.

Brown, J. S., Collins, A. & Duguid, P. (1989) Situated cognition and the culture of learning. *Educational Researcher* **18** (1), 32–42.

Bruner, J. (1986) *Actual Minds, Possible Worlds*. Harvard University Press, Cambridge, Mass.

Burns, S. (1992) Grading practice. *Nursing Times* **88** (1), 40–2.

Clamp, C. (1980) Learning through incidents. *Nursing Times* **76** (40), 1755–8.

Entwistle, N. (1998) Supporting students' frameworks for conceptual understanding: knowledge objects and their implications. In *Improving Student Learning: Improving Students as Learners* (C. Rust, ed.), pp. 206–14. Oxford Centre for Staff and Learning Development, Oxford.

Flanagan, J. C. (1954) The critical incident technique. *Psychological Bulletin* **5**, 327–58.

Fleming, N. D. (1995) *I'm different: not dumb. Modes of presentation (V.A.R.K.) in the tertiary classroom*. A paper given at the Higher Education Research And Development Society of Australasia (HERDSA), Rockhampton.

Hedlund, D. E., Furst, T. C. & Foley, K. T. (1989) A dialogue with self: the journal as an educational tool. *Journal of Humanistic Education and Development* 27, March, 105–13.

Holly, M.L. (1989) *Teacher Enquiry: Keeping a Personal Professional Journal*. Heinemann Educational Books, Portsmouth.

Jarvis, P. & Gibson, S. (1997) *The Teacher Practitioner in Nursing and Midwifery and Health Visiting*. Chapman & Hall, London.

Knowles, M. (1975) *Self Directed Learning*. Cambridge, New York.

Marton, F. & Säljö, R. (1997) Approaches to learning. In *The Experience of Learning: Implications for Teaching and Studying in Higher Education*, 2nd edn (F. Marton, D. Hounsell & N. Entwistle, eds), pp. 39–58. Scottish Academic Press, Edinburgh.

Mezirow, J. (1981) A critical theory of adult education and learning. *Adult Education* 32 (1), 3–24.

Miller, C. (1995) *Researching Professional Education: Learning Styles and Facilitating Reflection*. English National Board for Nursing, Midwifery and Health Visiting, London.

Revans, R. (1982) *The Origins and Growth of Action Learning*. Bratt Institut für Neues Learning, Harvestor.

Spouse, J. (1998a) *Understanding learning in the professional context: Five case studies of nurses from a pre-registration degree course*. Unpublished PhD thesis, University of Bath, pp. 94–9.

Spouse, J. (1998b) Scaffolding student learning in clinical practice. *Nurse Education Today* 18, 259–66.

Taylor, M. (1987) Self directed learning: more than meets the observer's eye. In *Appreciating Adults Learning: From the Learner's Perspective* (D. Boud & V. Griffin, eds), pp. 179–96. Kogan Page, London.

Tompkins, C. & McGraw, M-J. (1981) The negotiated learning contract. In *Developing Student Autonomy in Learning* (D. Boud, ed.) pp. 172–92. Kogan Page, London.

Tripp, D. (1993) *Critical Incidents in Teaching: Developing Professional Judgement*. Routledge, London.

Wertsch, J. & Stone, C.A (1979) A social interactional analysis of learning disabilities remediation. Paper presented at International Conference of Association for Children with Learning Disabilities, San Francisco. In *Everyday Cognition: Its Development in the Social Context* (B. Rogoff & J. Lave, eds). Springer, Cambridge, Mass, 1984.

Chapter 7

Supervision of Practice and the New National Health Service Quality Agenda

Liz Redfern with a contribution from David Robson

A hallmark of any profession is its collective desire to improve and move forward through research and contemplation so that lessons can be learnt from what has gone before. Seeking supervision about one's practice is now established as one form of this action learning, as the case studies in earlier chapters show. Whilst the case studies broadly illustrate the consequences for the individual participating in a supervisory relationship, the role of supervision in the wider quality agenda is yet to be determined as the NHS finds itself approaching the end of the twentieth century.

For me the following questions are raised by the case studies and the other chapters of this book:

- What evidence do the professions already using supervision in support of practice development have that it makes a difference, and if we have no evidence should we be extending the practice?
- Is the form of supervision that is derived from one used widely in counselling and social work appropriate for widespread use by all staff, including doctors? Does it fit the cultural makeup of all professions in health care?
- If supervision could be accepted by employers as a useful tool to help them meet quality targets, how much would it really cost to implement properly?
- Do these case studies represent a small minority of people who are practising supervision or is it now embedded in the culture of the professions represented here?
- How do we develop open and transparent quality systems when supervision is usually a confidential activity? Is it possible to create a safe space for professionals to reflect on their practice without it being

shrouded in secrecy? Should we expect employers to fund an activity where the content cannot be subjected to scrutiny and where the benefits to the organisation are unclear?

This chapter does not attempt to answer all these questions as some of them are unanswerable at this stage, but it attempts to set some of the questions in context and create a debate that is not about blindly accepting supervision as good, but about finding ways of defending its value in the day-to-day world of health care.

The extent to which finance drove and dominated the health care agenda to the exclusion of quality issues in the decade until 1997 was a universal concern frequently aired by health professionals whatever their nationality. One of the consequences of this type of policy in the UK has been the disinvestment in staffing structures and staff development opportunities which has severely reduced support structures and supervision opportunities for the professional workforce. Examples of this disinvestment include the dilution of the grade and skill mix of the non-medical workforce; the reduction in the amount of study leave and funding available for qualified professionals to keep themselves up to date; and inaccurate workforce planning leading to a reduction in the number of students needed to maintain the size of professional groups. These factors have all had an impact on the quality of care the National Health Service has been able to provide. In response to this lack of support from one's colleagues and professional management structures, the idea of supervision was seen by many as an acceptable alternative support structure and by others as a method of learning from experience. In fact supervision of practice is probably one of the most underrated forms of work-based learning, but we rarely sell it as such.

As I write this chapter the newspaper headlines warn the public of a nursing staffing crisis which is having a direct impact on the ability of NHS hospitals to admit and care for patients. Nurses are always a newsworthy subject but it would have been just as accurate to talk about a staffing crisis in the other smaller professional groups such as physiotherapists, radiographers, dieticians or pharmacists. This staffing crisis is a result of many factors, particularly the inability of some professions, such as nursing, to recruit people into the pre-registration programmes and the ability of others to retain staff within the NHS. These issues are not unique to the UK and are challenging managers within health services on a global scale. They all have an impact on the ability of a health service to provide quality care within a quality experience for the patient.

Concerns about falling standards of care in nursing were brought into sharp focus by the tragic events uncovered in the Clothier Report (Clothier *et al.* 1994) which examined the circumstances surrounding the death of children under the care of a nurse, Beverly Allitt. Bishop (1994) highlights how the Allitt inquiry, along with other criticisms of nursing, concentrated the minds of the nurses at the NHS executive who saw clinical supervision as being the first stage of evolving a mechanism to support high quality clinical care. This changing context for nursing formed a backdrop for the creation of health care policy that had considerable influence on the development of clinical supervision, which was seen by Yvonne Moores (Chief Nursing Officer for England) (Department of Health 1994) as fundamental to safeguarding standards, the development of professional expertise and the delivery of care. It is, of course, impossible to speculate whether having a system of clinical supervision in place would have prevented the actions of someone such as Beverly Allitt, or whether her actions would have been detected sooner.

Supervision was already a well accepted practice in midwifery, physiotherapy and occupational therapy. Nursing could be considered to be late in introducing the idea. However, the timeliness of an idea is just as important as its pedigree, and clinical supervision came at a time when nursing education was accepting the value of experiential learning (ENB 1992) and reflective practice as a legitimate form of professional learning. Reflective practice is also the common link between clinical supervision and the use of profiles or portfolios to provide evidence of experiential learning. The statutory and professional bodies, the nursing press and the policy makers at the NHS Executive all seemed to be in agreement that these 'softer' approaches to learning should be encouraged and supported by the nursing establishment. However, the employers were not always convinced (Rudd & Wolsey 1997). Some money was available, through a bidding process, to set up local clinical supervision strategies and train clinical supervisors, but the employers had to bear the cost of releasing staff from the workplace to participate in clinical supervision at a time of great cost pressures on Trust budgets. It was difficult to persuade Trust boards that introducing clinical supervision would give value for money and provide added value by improving rates of staff sickness and absence, improving the recruitment and retention of staff, reducing the number of patient complaints and contributing to the Trust risk management strategy. To fulfil all of these aims would be a tall order for any model of professional development.

There is anecdotal evidence and an intuitive feeling from enthusiasts that clinical supervision does provide a restorative function (Proctor 1991) for professionals who are dealing with and working in stressful situations. However, it is recognised that there needs to be a more systematic evaluation of the link between clinical supervision and clinical outcomes (Butterworth *et al.* 1996). Following a workshop in early 1995 to explore which assessment tools would be effective in the evaluation of clinical supervision, a decision was made to establish a national evaluation exercise in nursing (Butterworth 1997). A very readable report of the evaluation study was published in the *Nursing Times* in October 1997 and so the details are not repeated here. Although the study did find numerous benefits to be gained for those participating in clinical supervision, it did not satisfy hard-line managers about the link between the experience of participating in clinical supervision and improved patient outcomes. The study did show that:

- Seventy per cent of all participants receiving clinical supervision were overwhelmingly positive about the experience
- Results from a general health questionnaire suggested that those not receiving clinical supervision were more likely to score highly – a sign of increased psychological distress
- There was an increase in emotional exhaustion and depersonalisation during a period when no clinical supervision was available. Once clinical supervision was introduced, the levels stabilised and decreased in some cases
- When clinical supervision was withdrawn there was significant reduction in job satisfaction

The study did not make the direct link between the presence of clinical supervision and patient outcomes, but it would be very difficult to do this in view of all the variables involved. The outcomes it did show were about staff feeling less stressed and enjoying their jobs more, and the title of the published study, 'It's good to talk', reflected this (Butterworth *et al.* 1997). At a time when the health service is facing a recruitment and retention crisis, it would seem from this evaluation study that providing clinical supervision as an employer may well lead to staff staying with you because they are being provided with a supportive mechanism to deal with the day-to-day stresses of working in the health service.

Although completed before the outcome of the study, Fowler (1996), in a review of the literature about how clinical supervision in nursing has been implemented, states that the literature appears largely to consider clinical supervision as a 'good thing', and that the counselling model dominates. The psychological methodology underpinning the Butterworth study brought criticism from those who were already convinced that clinical supervision as a process was too much in the grip of counselling models of supervision (Rudd & Wolsey 1997), which may not bring appropriate outcomes as perceived by the health service. They cite Bernard & Goodyear (1992) who argue that as long as supervision remains anchored in the theories of therapy it will never develop its own scientific base. In other words, they believe, there is no science of supervision.

Rudd & Wolsey (1997) go on to argue that to justify the significant expense of supervision it will be essential to demonstrate to the purchasers of health care how it benefits the patients and the service, and to demonstrate to the practitioners how it will help them perform and survive in a constantly changing job market. Even with a change of government since Rudd & Wolsey wrote their article, the NHS still has to balance limited resources with increasing demands. Any new money injected into the NHS by the Government is still linked with demonstrable targets of achievement which continue to put pressure on staff to perform. Although the enthusiasts for clinical supervision have ensured that it has had wide exposure to nursing staff, it is probably fair to say that the practice of clinical supervision has not yet gained wide understanding or acceptance by all nurses. Five years on it is certainly not embedded in nursing practice or culture. Clinical supervision is at an interesting time in its short history, and nursing needs to find ways of defending its usefulness in ways that are understood and valued by health service managers. The case studies in this book clearly show the benefits that supervision of practice can bring to individuals, but they generate little evidence of how they might help a trust or a primary care group to meet the latest political imperatives of reducing waiting lists, controlling prescribing budgets or introducing evidence-based practice to meet the clinical effectiveness agenda.

In 1997 health policy changed course and through the publication of the White Paper 'The new NHS: modern, dependable' (Department of Health 1997) there was an attempt to put the quality agenda back into health care. In the White Paper and its subsequent document, 'A first class service: quality in the new NHS' (Department of Health 1998a) the Government made it clear that there would be a statutory duty for quality on the part of each NHS hospital and community Trust and primary care group. This would be achieved through the introduction of clinical governance. Clinical governance is a framework through which NHS organisations are accountable for continuously improving the quality of their services and for safeguarding high standards of care.

Black (1998) sees clinical governance as an extension of the concept of corporate governance that had previously sought to bring in robust financial and administrative quality systems to ensure that an organisation was properly run. To Black, the extension of the concept of corporate governance to clinical matters was one of the most fundamental and radical of the Government's proposals within the White Paper. One of the driving principles of the White Paper is to ensure that the NHS provides a national service which prevents inequalities between the type and quality of service that people might experience just because of where they live. The new model marries clinical judgement with clear national standards. Such standards will be set through national service frameworks and through a

National Institute for Clinical Excellence which was launched on 1 April 1999. Standards will be delivered locally through the new system of clinical governance, lifelong learning and professional self-regulation. The achievement of these standards will be monitored and audited locally and through the Commission for Health Improvement.

The document (Department of Health 1998a) expands on each of these by saying that:

- Clinical governance will be the process by which each part of the NHS quality assures its clinical decisions
- Lifelong learning will give NHS staff the tools of knowledge to offer the most modern, effective and high quality care to patients
- Professional self-regulation will allow the professions to more openly account for how standards are set and enforced. Modern professional self-regulation will play a fuller part in the early identification of possible lapses in clinical quality

Supervision is certainly a tool of lifelong learning and, it can be argued, is a characteristic of a profession that is self-regulating. It is with this agenda in mind that we should be arguing the value of supervision with employers rather than the benefits of how it makes staff feel. According to Butterworth & Woods (1999) participating in clinical supervision in an active way is a clear example of how to exercise individual responsibility under clinical supervision.

Clinical governance is about a framework of activity that reaches into every part of the Trust or primary care group, and it will test the effectiveness of the organisation, the staff and the clinical practices as Fig. 7.1 shows.

Clinical governance can only be achieved through the people in the organisation, which brings me to the final document, 'Working together : securing a quality workforce' (Department of Health 1998b). This human resource framework document has the following statement as one of its strategic aims:

> '...we must ensure that we have a quality workforce, in the right numbers, with the right skills and diversity, organised in the right way, to deliver the Government's service objectives for health and social care.'

The ability to recruit a workforce in the right numbers is a labour market issue, but the ability of an organisation or profession to retain a workforce is a people management issue. The human resource framework recognises the need to set up systems which allow and enable employees to

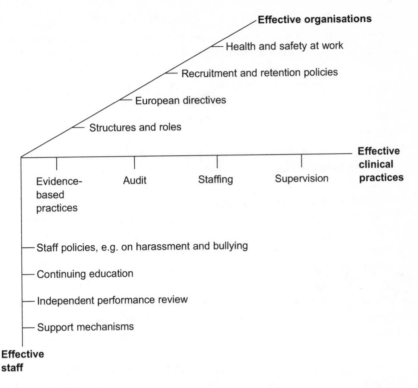

Fig. 7.1   Creating clinical governance.

understand how they can contribute to the organisation and to receive regular constructive feedback about how they are doing and how they need to develop further. Effective appraisal and mentoring systems should be at the heart of any human resource framework if quality performance is going to be recognised and poor performance is going to be addressed.

So what contribution could a supervision model of professional development make to this new agenda about quality, standards, clinical governance, lifelong learning, professional self-regulation and developing an effective workforce? Could it be a model that is picked up by all healthcare professions that have to operate within the concept of clinical governance? The wide range of non-medical professions represented within the case studies in this book would suggest that it could.

If clinical governance can only be achieved through the people in the organisation, I believe that will require organisations to rewrite the psychological contract they have with staff. What I mean by this is that staff need to experience their employing organisation as a place that nurtures their skills and qualities by rewarding and valuing them, rather than destroying their motivation and commitment by demanding more and more of them until burnout occurs. Lifelong learning can be an organisational characteristic as well as a personal characteristic. An organisation that learns from its mistakes and grows from them enables and allows staff to admit when things have gone wrong. An organisation that has a punishment culture only encourages individuals to hide mistakes away. The culture of an organisation can stifle creativity if new ideas brought in by new staff or those returning from a course are belittled by those who have tried it before, and because it did not work for them do not expect it will work for anyone else.

An organisational culture of lifelong learning encourages its employees to develop a sense of self-respect because they are trusted to use their judgement and their internal supervisor in making decisions (Senge 1990). In this type of culture the organisation has an adult-to-adult relationship with their employees, rather than a parent and child relationship.

Good supervision, according to Daloz (1987), is about the supervisor balancing the three elements of challenge, support and vision with the supervisee. His triangular model has been adapted by Northcott (1996) to show the effect on the individual when these elements are present within any supervisory relationship, including that within clinical supervision. The model could equally be applied to a workforce or profession in an organisational sense.

Any supervisory relationship using the Daloz elements encourages the growth of the person being supervised. This element of growth usually includes the individual eventually being able to provide their own internal supervisor, mentor, auditor, so creating real self-regulation. The supervisor enables the practitioner to reflect on their practice and to develop the skill of looking at it in an objective way, almost as a non-participant observer. Eventually the practitioner can learn to do this for themselves and the need for an external supervisor diminishes and may disappear. At the same time, of course, the practitioner is learning more about the way they practise and begins to understand what motivates them to practise in a particular way as well as identifying where they need to update themselves or approach a situation differently. The majority of health professionals are experiential learners and their pre-qualifying programmes depend on this fact by using some type of clinical placement as a teaching and learning method. Supervision of practice capitalises on the experiential learning method and so a model of lifelong learning can be developed which combines the need to learn from our experience as well as satisfying any unconnected lust for knowledge. As the case studies show, supervision is an approach that can develop a habit of lifelong learning as well as developing an internal auditor of standards of practice and self-regulation.

Self-regulation and professional self-regulation are not separate concepts. The nursing, midwifery and medical professions have enjoyed the freedom of professional self-regulation for decades and now the concept is under real political scrutiny for the first time. The public scandals of the high death rate of babies and children undergoing heart surgery in Bristol (1998) and the seeming inability of the United Kingdom Central Council (UKCC) to remove a rapist from the nursing register (1997) has thrown the existing mechanisms for professional self-regulation into sharp media, public and political focus. The introduction of clinical governance is seen by some as the last chance for the professions to prove themselves worthy of the responsibility for self-regulation. Rather like lifelong learning, self-regulation can be seen as an organisational or professional or individual characteristic. From whatever perspective, it depends upon a set of values and beliefs being present to create a culture where:

- There is an understanding of right and wrong, and what makes the difference between the two
- There is the support to ask difficult questions and not be afraid of the answers
- There is the courage to admit you might have been wrong
- There is the strength to identify and deal with poor performance in a constructive way
- There is the willingness to make difficult decisions in the face of popular opinion

What do we know already about the way individuals, organisations or professional groups set their internal standards? Bosk (1977) argues that each occupational group possesses its own morality and can possess a collective conscience which may serve the solidarity of the group, at some cost to the larger society. He studied in some depth surgeons in an American teaching hospital and collected data on how surgeons recognised, defined, punished and denied failure, using methods of social control over their peers. It makes interesting reading, particularly in the light of the Bristol scandal. In sociological terms, social control can have two distinct meanings (Janowitz 1976). It can refer to a group's ability to regulate itself on its own initiative or it can refer to the coercive means at a group's disposal to discipline individuals. Health professionals are socialised into their occupational group culture in insidious ways and are kept within the group's control, through their control of his/her career path. This is particularly true for doctors.

The coercive version of social control militates against the creation of a culture where openness and learning are the norm.

The document 'A first class service' (Department of Health 1998a) states that professional self-regulation has to be earned, and to justify this freedom the professions must be openly accountable for the standards they set and the way they are enforced. In other words, the heroic culture which denies there is a problem or pushes it underground in the hope that the problem will not be discovered has no place in the modern, dependable NHS. The new quality agenda is demanding a major cultural change for everyone involved in health care, from the professionals to the patients. That cultural change will need strong leadership from the Chief Executive at the top of the organisation and from those who lead the professional and occupational groups. Major cultural change takes a long time and needs to be supported with mechanisms to encourage a 'bottom-up' approach. Could one of those mechanisms be the models of supervision illustrated through the case studies, or evolved versions of those models?

As the case studies show, supervision is a way of enabling individual practitioners to learn about their own practice through reflection, with the intention of improving and developing it to the benefit of the patient/client. This type of discovery learning may confirm that their practice is of a good enough standard or it may confirm that further theoretical or practical work needs to be done by the practitioner in order to improve the standard of practice. This type of discovery, rea-lisation and critical self-appraisal only usually occurs in an atmosphere of trust and mutual respect. During supervision this is usually estab-lished over a period of time between the members of the group and their facilitator, or between the supervisee and the supervisor in a one-to-one relationship. In the nursing model of clinical supervision, the relation is usually within a context of confidentiality and disconnected from any managerial or disciplinary processes. Establishing the security of knowing that whatever you say within a clinical supervision setting will not be held in evidence against you has always been important as a baseline when setting up clinical supervision protocols. Culturally, it seems it is very difficult for nursing to tolerate poor care and use it as a learning opportunity. Part of me thinks that is quite right if nurses are to act as the patients' advocate, but on the other hand a punitive, unfor-giving culture encourages mistakes to be hidden rather than exposed and used positively or denied as Bosk (1977) showed. Hiding and deny-ing poor practice is a dangerous and risky business when most of the time nurses, doctors and the professions allied to medicine are dealing with people at their most vulnerable. Neal (1998) explains that the UKCC sees clinical supervision as part of a framework for managing risk. It sees supervision as providing the final link between the theory of accountability and the pragmatics of practice. Supervision should be seen as taking its place in a wider framework of activities that are designed to underpin the delivery of high quality clinical services. A way of helping to guarantee that the quality agenda is delivered to the public and the politicians is by ensuring effective communication between the key components of clinical risk management, clinical audit, practice and professional development and research.

The concern nurses have about using clinical supervision as a means of exploring poor practice also relates to the way clinical supervision sessions are recorded. This is an area of concern that nurses turn to the UKCC for advice about. Neal (1998) reported that the UKCC's legal adviser holds the view that documents developed by virtue of employment are owned by the employer. She goes on to explain that this means that if there is a contractual requirement for the employee to participate in clinical supervision then the records are owned by the employer. But if an employer merely encourages the employee to participate, then any records made are probably in the possession of the employee. This begs the question as to what happens if there is no contractual obligation to participate but the employer provides you with the time and the resources to do so. Where does all this legalistic approach take us if we are trying to create a different culture, one where processes are open and transparent and clinical supervision is about learning from practice and using that learning as a springboard for change?

Nursing has had its difficulties in implementing clinical supervision because of scarce resources and the cynicism of some practitioners that 'We have always done it and there is no need to change now'. At least it has been successful in small pockets of the profession. Where staff have participated, and the clinical supervisors have been trained and skilled, staff have reported how they have found it a supportive activity. This book shows examples of how the principle has been applied in other professions, but should supervision be rolled out across all professions as part of the clinical governance agenda? How would it be received by doctors?

In putting together the contents of this book Jenny Spouse and I were keen to connect into the opinions of medical colleagues and through a contact we are able to include some reflections from David Robson, who is an NHS consultant physician. These are his personal reflections:

'...perhaps the most important point I want to make is that, as a consultant in the NHS, there is no established reflective or supervisory framework in which one operates. I would agree with the points made earlier in this chapter, that there would need to be a substantial cultural shift in order to create one and to ensure it works in a meaningful way. The majority of the case studies within this book refer to a situation where a more experienced professional is supervising a student or less experienced professional and concepts of mutual and co-supervision do not occur. Any framework developed for medical staff would need to take this into account, particularly if there is to be a positive move forward on the issue of clinical governance. It would be too easy for any system of supervision to become a method of 'sloganising' the political differences between or within groups. This could become a way of dealing with the tensions and anxieties caused by an attempt to confront the appropriateness or otherwise of the care we offer to patients. We cannot ignore the political and social purpose of supervision, although it is sometimes difficult to understand how one-to-one interactions can be seen in a social and political context. In order to do that, it seems that we may have to ask some uncomfortable questions about the stated and unstated purposes of supervision and where they fit with the individual and organisational motives.

'The case studies have stimulated me to think about what opportunities there might be for me to receive or participate in supervision. My personal situation begins to illustrate some of the difficulties in establishing a common system.

'My clinical duties cover cardiology, intensive care and general acute medicine on my admission days. It is immediately evident from this list that my spread of work is far from homogeneous. At one end of the spectrum are a range of highly technical procedures and decisions about which there may be only one or two other people in the Trust with enough experience to enter into a meaningful dialogue with. To take another specific example. There are only three people who are employed by the Trust, of whom I am one, with the appropriate skills and knowledge to carry out coronary angiograms. If I have a problem in this area, there are limited opportunities to review my performance. Recognising this, we have set up a permanent audit of coronary angiography so that every case has its complications recorded and we publish the results monthly within the department. How effective this system is is a matter for speculation. In particular I am doubtful how effective it would remain if there were conflicts between the key figures.

'My work in intensive care also provides similar examples of the need to make complex decisions which very few people are qualified to take. These skills are used alongside others where it is possible to find other members of the team with equivalent or superior skills. An example of this would be face-to-face contact with patients and their families. Here there exists considerable scope for discussion as to how issues should be handled and for a review between the doctor and the nurse about how the interaction proceeded. Another example of note is the area of complex decision making about whether to withdraw or continue with therapy. Although this is an area where my experience counts, I find it difficult to consider myself an expert. All those involved in the care will have a view, and the challenge is to find a framework for mutual expression of those views, whilst permitting decisions to be taken. Finally from my own practice there is the area of general medicine. The sheer breadth and variation of problems that come in through the door mean that no one can truly be considered to be an expert: at best we are gifted amateurs. This is often an area of my work where it is clear that sometimes the juniors in the team may know more than the seniors.

'The spotlight seems to be on doctors as a result of the political quality agenda which has been fed by the events in Bristol. Signposting the absence of a supervisory framework in these circumstances seems to over-simplify the issues. To put it simply, far more children were dying than would have seemed appropriate. Having said that, the failure was clearly much wider than the cardiac surgeons and the chief executive who have found themselves in the public eye. All the babies who died were referred by paediatric cardiologists. The quality of the investigations may have had some bearing on the surgical outcome, and as a physician it is always possible to stop referring patients to a surgeon whose performance or competencies you judge to be inappropriately stretched by the particular case in question. The point here is that unless cultural attitudes to supervision change in such a way that it becomes a way of life for all the health professions, the NHS will continue to be open to the kind of problem experienced at Bristol.

'Failure on that scale is, I believe, a corporate failure, rather than just a failure of individuals in the system. I feel very strongly that any model of supervision will need to run through the practice of medicine from top to bottom and side to side. Encompassing all professions and all grades will be the only way to ensure a cultural change in our hospitals and health care organisations. Making the activity culture wide will prevent the cultural isolation of various groups which facilitated the kind of situation that arose within the Bristol case. This widespread cultural change is the real challenge; whether it is too great a challenge only time will tell.'

Despite David's obvious commitment to finding ways of improving his practice, his reflections clearly show that developing frameworks of supervision to spread across all settings and professions within health care is not going to be easy. His concerns about where he might find co-supervision for some of his specialist work will be shared by any practitioner working in a highly specialised field. Most models of supervision assume that the expertise of the supervisor will be found within the same organisation as the professional seeking supervision, but this may not apply in the case of the highly specialised practitioner. Going outside the organisation for supervision on some aspects of practice may not be practical and it will incur additional cost implications. But is it the role of the supervisor to provide subject expertise, or is it about providing facilitative skills to help the supervisee reflect on their practice and solve the problems for themselves?

The opposite problem to where a specialist might seek supervision from if they are the only expert in their organisation occurs for general practitioners who are needed to be expert generalists. Do they seek supervision from several directions to cover their clinical decision making on such a wide range of diseases, conditions and ailments? Just as Trusts have a responsibility to establish mechanisms for implementing clinical governance, so primary care groups (PCGs) have the same duty to ensure clinical governance is in place. PCGs are new health care organisations made up of elected GPs, community nurses, social workers, lay members and a non-executive director from the overseeing health authority. GPs often consider themselves to be independent contractors who are only accountable to their patients for the quality of their clinical decision making. The concept of clinical governance, which will require a collective understanding and commitment to providing, amongst other things, evidence-based care, is an interesting one when applied to independent contractor status. In many ways PCGs are virtual organisations comprising a range of different types and sizes of GP practices. This makes it much more difficult, but not impossible, to use strategies that might be applicable to a large single-site hospital Trust. These issues will pose real challenges to PCGs if they are to implement mechanisms, systems and structures to support the clinical governance agenda. It will be necessary for PCGs to deal with some of the basics such as how they get their constituent GP practices on board with these issues before opportunities to introduce ideas about how mechanisms such as supervision might make a contribution to the quality agenda.

So where does all this lead us? We believe that the theoretical chapters in this book, combined with the stories of those who have recounted so honestly their experiences, begin to provide evidence that the supervision of professional practice has a positive contribution to make to the new NHS quality agenda. It is important that we quickly gain insight and knowledge about how that contribution will be assessed so that we can present rational arguments to the new quality gatekeepers in terms they will understand about how supervision deserves to be one tool in the clinical governance survival kit.

References

Bernard, J.M. & Goodyear, R.K. (1992) *Fundamentals of Clinical Supervision.* Allyn & Bacon, Needham Heights, NY.

Bishop, V. (1994) Clinical supervision for an accountable profession. *Nursing Times* **90** (39), 27–8.

Black, N. (1998) Clinical governance: fine words or action. *British Medical Journal* **316** (24 January), 297–8.

Bosk, C.L. (1977) *Forgive and Remember: Managing Medical Failure*. Penguin, London.

Butterworth, A. (1997) Clinical supervision: a hornet's nest? Or honey pot? *Nursing Times* **93** (44), 26.

Butterworth, A. & Woods, D. (1999) Clinical governance and clinical supervision; working together to ensure safe and accountable practice. University of Manchester briefing paper.

Butterworth, A., Bishop, V. & Carson, J. (1996) First steps towards evaluating clinical supervision in nursing and health visiting. 1. Theory, policy and practice development. A review. *Journal of Clinical Nursing* **5**, 127–32.

Clothier, C., Macdonald, C. A. & Shaw, D. A. (1994) *The Allitt Inquiry*. HMSO, London.

Daloz, L.A. (1987) *Effective Teaching and Mentoring*. Jossey Bass, San Francisco.

Department of Health (1994) CNO letter 94(5) *Clinical Supervision for the Nursing and Midwifery Professions*. HMSO, London.

Department of Health (1997) The new NHS: modern, dependable. HMSO, London.

Department of Health (1998a) A First Class Service: quality in the new NHS. HMSO, London.

Department of Health (1998b) Working together: securing a quality workforce for the NHS. HMSO, London.

English National Board for Nursing, Midwifery and Health Visiting (1992) *Framework for Continuing Professional Education*. ENB, London.

Fowler, J. (1996) The organisation of clinical supervision within the nursing profession: a review of the literature. *Journal of Advanced Nursing* **23**, 471–8.

Neal, K. (1998) A framework for managing risk. *Nursing Times Learning Curve* **1** (12), 4–5.

Northcott, N. (1996) Supervise to grow. *Nursing Management* **2** (10).

Proctor, B. (1991) On being a trainer. In *Training and Supervision for Counselling in Action* (W. Dryden & B. Thorne, eds). Sage, London.

Rudd, L. & Wolsey, P. (1997) Clinical supervision: a hornet's nest? Or honey pot? *Nursing Times* **93** (44), 25.

Senge, P.M. (1990) *The Fifth Discipline: The Art and Practice of the Learning Organisation*. Century Business, London.

Index